I0693365

EGO OF THE WARRIOR

ROB SIRSTINS

BALBOA.PRESS

A DIVISION OF HAY HOUSE

Balboa Press books may be ordered through booksellers or by contacting:

Balboa Press
A Division of Hay House
1663 Liberty Drive
Bloomington, IN 47403
www.balboapress.com
844-682-1282

Because of the dynamic nature of the Internet, any web addresses or links contained in this book may have changed since publication and may no longer be valid. The views expressed in this work are solely those of the author and do not necessarily reflect the views of the publisher, and the publisher hereby disclaims any responsibility for them.

The author of this book does not dispense medical advice or prescribe the use of any technique as a form of treatment for physical, emotional, or medical problems without the advice of a physician, either directly or indirectly. The intent of the author is only to offer information of a general nature to help you in your quest for emotional and spiritual well-being. In the event you use any of the information in this book for yourself, which is your constitutional right, the author and the publisher assume no responsibility for your actions.

Any people depicted in stock imagery provided by Getty Images are models, and such images are being used for illustrative purposes only.
Certain stock imagery © Getty Images.

Print information available on the last page.

ISBN: 978-1-9822-5981-5 (sc)
ISBN: 978-1-9822-5982-2 (hc)
ISBN: 978-1-9822-5983-9 (e)

Library of Congress Control Number: 2020923688

Balboa Press rev. date: 12/10/2021

Ego Of The Warrior

CONTENTS

Introduction ix

I 1
II 11
III 21
IV 32
V 42
VI 52
VII 62
VIII 72
IX 81
X 89
XI 100
XII 108
XIII 118

Closing Remarks 127
Appreciation 129
References 131

INTRODUCTION

There is a magical power deep within you, found only if you are willing to search and uncover your truth. Perhaps it has been calcified under immense pain, confusion, and heartbreak, and the thought of venturing once again to rediscover what is buried deep may seem frightening. Very few take this journey. However, you picked this book up, so that isn't you. You are ready to keep moving forward, to change, to become. You are ready to heal that which was once broken and to strengthen that which was once weak.

Once this power is discovered and attained, one must step into it with all their might without hesitation, embarrassment, or fear to honor the gifts that have been bestowed upon you.

You will then uphold this power unapologetically, fearlessly, and without shame. For this is your power, specific to you only. To be willing to shine and bring forth into the world your light and your story. Then to help others see what is wrought within themselves. Only if you are willing to do the work and take the path of shedding off the old and stepping into who you truly are will you become a warrior. The path of the Warrior is the conscious, physical, emotional, mental, and spiritual fight to heal, find center, and become your true divine self. It is a battle. It is a war of attrition we fight against ourselves, our stories, and our minds. It is more challenging than anything else we can possibly face in this life.

Although I attribute this process to that of a Warrior, the goal is not to become resistant but to gain acceptance, allowance, and faith.

This process enables us to accept our past, regardless of what has happened, because nothing can be done back there, but only here and now.

We learn to allow what is to come, rather than stress continuously of controlling that which cannot be controlled.

We grow in faith that we can and will heal from our past and become empowered more than we can imagine for our present and our future.

Throughout this book, I will challenge you to look at yourself, your patterns, and your stories through a different lens. I will show you a close and personal view of my failures, as well as my self-incriminating way of thinking. I will also show you how I decided to be a victim of my circumstances no longer, to no longer live on my knees from an indoctrinated belief system I fell into long before I could walk.

I will challenge you to step out of the darkness with the power and strength needed to see your true, higher self.

It is time to put down the facades dictated by insecurities and trauma. It is time to rise and become the sole operator of your fragile life.

Every person put on this earth has a higher purpose of fulfilling the potential of being who they are meant to be, but too many people never realize their purpose because they are too afraid.

Before I go on, I want you to understand as the reader that I'm talking with you as if you were sitting next to me. That when I say we, I know that you picked up my book because we share something in common.

Sometimes, we find ourselves being triggered and spiraling down dark holes for reasons we don't yet understand. All we know is that we have pain, we've held on to emotional memories, and some of us are carrying weight that exceeds our breaking point. Some of us have found an escape, a way to temper the pain, such as physical activity, creative arts, or meditation. But for those of us dealing with something much deeper, darker, more painful, that is all those outlets do—temper.

I would like you to come on a close and personal journey with me as I share the most traumatic and life-altering situations I've experienced. How I moved from being a victim of abandonment and racism to a man of humble power and understanding. From being a casualty of the whirlwind of emotions inside me, and the irrational decisions I made because of them, to creating a masterpiece from my chaos and pain.

I hope to do more than motivate you by moving you into action and help you create a path to find your own divine power and calling. I hope to help you change your perspective and your toxic way of thinking.

I'll take you through the process I went through to find myself for the first time. For some, it may be for a second or third time as this process is meant to expand us into becoming who we truly are meant to be, and that takes time. Through my philosophies, I hope to help give you a different opportunity to move into yourself while removing old and damaging expectations, and helping you to realize you are the creator of every one of your limitations.

I realize this path is not for everyone, nor do I claim this is the "be all, cure-all." This book is about the path of my journey, my pain, my darkness and how I came out on the other side, rather than another statistic of suicide.

If you are looking for another way to heal or just another perspective, take a look at my life and the toxic thinking I was committed to for so long.

I am not a psychologist or therapist. I am simply a battle-riddled man who found his power through the journey you are about to embark on.

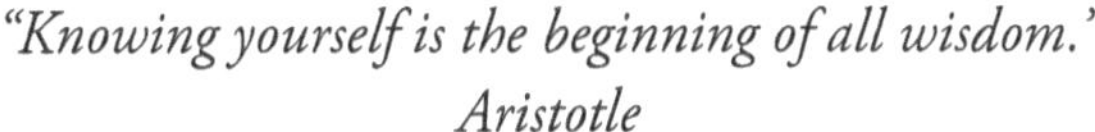

"Knowing yourself is the beginning of all wisdom."
Aristotle

In early October of 1981, I was born to a 17-year-old girl in the Maricopa Hospital in Phoenix, Arizona. My mother was young in her years and badly affected with personal and emotional problems. I was told she battled drug addiction, promiscuity, and severe mental challenges.

In my short three months with my biological mother, my four-year-old sister and I had a small taste of her chaotic world.

I never knew anything about my biological father. I assume that he was a larger man, as my mother stood at only five feet. I believe their relationship was a one-time occurrence since there is no real record of him, which invigorates my ongoing search of where I come from, trying to answer the forever question plaguing so many who have been wards of the state, growing up in foster care, or lucky enough to be adopted as I was.

My sister had obviously a much better recollection than I did during those few months before we were given up to foster care then quickly adopted.

I was told our mother would leave us for days at a time, in a one-room apartment with only my very young sister to care for me. There was no food left in the fridge, nor ready breast milk in a bottle, or clean clothes nicely folded for us to change into. She would vanish with no comforting words of when she would return.

My sister took on the role of the mother the best she could, caring for me and consoling me to the best of her four-year-old capabilities.

Before I was born, my mother would take my sister to the local grocery stores and taught her to distract the grocery store clerk so my mother could steal food. Because of this, my sister was able to sneak into the local grocery store every now and then to gather the food that she and I needed when our mother was absent.

Upon my mother's return, strung out from whatever her choice of drug was, she'd usually be accompanied by a man. They would have sex on the very same bed where my sister and I rested.

For the first three months of my life, this was my ordinary world. Chaos. Decades later, I finally came to the understanding of why those first few months played such an integral part of my life and how they affected me all the way until adulthood.

Why was I so fucking angry all the time? Pessimistic, distrusting, insecure, and anxious? I finally realized I had developed reactive attachment disorder, or RAD (Smith, 2018).

There are extensive cases that show children who fail to establish a strong bond with their mother or caretaker develop RAD. Cases range in severity, with symptoms including emotional instability, lack of self-confidence, anger, control issues, and trust. I battled with these symptoms, as well as feeling alone and unsafe.

I didn't really relate to others as I grew up for many obvious and not so obvious reasons. This is common for children who are abused, live in and out of foster care, are taken away from their parents, or were abandoned (Smith, 2018).

I never connected with my birth mother or father or cemented a bond built of trust and confidence as other newborn babies do. This was just the start of my blundering young life.

Luckily, my sister and I were eventually given to wonderful foster parents who eventually adopted us. We became part of a loving family with three older siblings. Even though this new environment was accepting of us and gave us the life that we could have only dreamed of, the trauma didn't stop there. Outside the walls of our home was a society that contrasted the nurturing space found within.

We all have setbacks, heartbreaks, failures, defeats, and traumas. Some people put these memories in the loss section of the brain and do their best to move on the only way they know how, by shifting into survival mode to make it through each day. That's what I did. I was not equipped with the knowledge or power to even know there were avenues that would allow me to grow and heal. Like so many of us, I just thought I had a permanent wound, left to scab over and get ripped back off from time to time.

What a fucking way to live. That was precisely how I lived my life well into my mid-30s. I lived the life of a man driven by anger, pain, confusion, and my closest friend, darkness.

I kept all of those yet unidentified emotions pent up inside me. But I was able to channel them all through my body, excelling in every sport I participated in. The fields and courts were the only places where I ever found solace growing up.

I was blessed with a pair of invisible wings that took me higher and faster than most any other kids around, but no amount of success I earned was enough to completely heal the void where my confidence was supposed to be or give me the ability to trust enough to be at peace with my surroundings. Playing sports was just a way to temper the pain, while my social reality outside of sports was where I never found happiness or freedom. I was a black boy with curly hair growing up in a very white society that had a very one-dimensional way of thinking.

In elementary school, I wasn't accepted among my peers or their parents. I was bullied, beaten, and made fun of. Usually, I spent most of those days running around my mother's daycare. The kids she tended to always accepted me more than the kids at school.

Because my peers at school didn't include me, I probably should have not accepted them, right? Even though my parents tried their best to teach me to be understanding, these were the very conversations I had in my head. I was still so confused and not able to make sense of why I was dealing with all these horrible feelings of rejection and sadness all of the time.

I thought this way for a long time. These thoughts never became lighter, and my internal, mental self-persecution only became more rampant. The world hated me, so I loathed me.

Isn't it amazing how impactful our early childhood years can be and the consequences that follow because of them? I spent most of my life searching for external validation to find self-love, acceptance, equality, and a desire to live.

I thwarted off any chance of believing in who I was and having the self-awareness of what I was most deserving. I became enthralled with a story and a program laid before me as soon as I could conceptualize my surroundings. I unwillingly chose to believe I was unworthy. That black would never be as good as white, and because of this belief, my limitations were outstanding.

It was as though a gray cloud would follow me around wherever I went, a constant reminder I was never good enough, attractive enough, or equal among those with white skin.

I heard the word *nigger* regularly, either directed ragefully towards me or under one's breath as they sheepishly walked past me.

My story could be told in the sense of how, especially in my younger years, I created an immovable beast of a man that tore down and conquered each feat one by one, but this isn't that type of story. I could go on to tell you how great of an athlete it made me by helping me obtain my one and only dream, but that dream was never realized. I could share that through my rage and anger, my story helped me become a millionaire by the time I was 25—then again, I would be lying.

This story is a walk through every significant traumatic event I have experienced. Rather than propelling me forward because of my grit, it almost killed me by a self-inflicted bullet to the head.

So, in turn, because of what I experienced, I created an indestructible shield of ego, and it set me on the course of absolute disloyalty to myself. Just so I could fit in and never have to be bullied again.

As I passed through junior high school, I began to be more accepted. I was a lone crusader—only two other students were black, and they were fraternal twins. With the rise of hip hop and music channels, I was able to see what it was like to be black outside my community. I felt I owed allegiance to the culture, even though I was as far away from the culture as one could be.

I did my best to be what I thought a young black man was supposed to be and was supposed to act. I was the same black kid you saw on television: the tough guy when I needed to be (even though I was scared shitless most of my adolescent years), the charming, loud, funny guy (even though I think I was just pretty much loud), then the athlete. Having first dunked a basketball in eighth grade and breaking track records as a freshman, the stereotype of a talented black athlete was one I proudly fulfilled. I surged ahead of the pack, outperforming peers at my home school and across the school district.

Although I was more accepted in junior high, bigotry was still ever-present.

I was always reminded by the "schools on the other side of the track" that I was a "whitewashed traitor."

In all reality, I would've given anything to go to those schools to feel like I belonged and not always reminded I was so different at home.

Stringing from my confusing young years and even through a large part of my adulthood, I wanted to be white. I tried to fit in and be respected. Rather than be judged immediately for the color of my skin, I wanted them to take a chance on me and get to know me. I didn't have a tribe at home who looked like me and who could empathize with my troubles and grant me answers to my questions.

I wanted to be looked at for who I was rather than judged by the preconceived notions of who others expected me to be from mainstream media. All the while, I had no idea who I was or who I wanted to become, and as time went on, my confusion only intensified.

I will continue to circle back to my story throughout this book. But one thing I wish I would've learned at such a young age is the ability to know self-love and accept my true self, or at least knowledge of the path to find those divine attributes.

When we're young, we are always asked by adults what we want to be when we grow up, and we rattle off things like doctor, lawyer, an athlete, but hardly we are ever asked WHO do we want to be? *Who* is the kind of man you want to be? *Who* is the type of woman you want to be? We never took the time to envision the *who*, only the *what*. Even until now, some of us have never questioned *who* we are because we have been so busy concerning ourselves only with the *what*.

Let's break this down a bit and get ready to answer some tough questions. Answer these honestly and openly, be vulnerable with yourself; lying to yourself will only hinder the process. These are interesting questions to ask and questions I'm not sure too many would like to answer publicly.

Are you currently happy with the person you have become?

What loads are you carrying that are inhibiting you from you?

Have you become a victim of your traumas as I had?

And by becoming the victim, have you become the very same creator of your pain by projecting it on others, passing along the very same cycle which was passed down to you? Or have you become what you have desperately needed to survive?

Have you become a chameleon in your career, your social settings, and with your family without even realizing it? Have you suffered a complete loss of identity? Are you living a life dictated by fear of being seen? Are you living the way you felt others wanted or even needed you to be? Do you ignore what your heart implores you to become?

Or do you feel you have stepped into yourself or have begun to do so?

If so, do you defend and honor yourself by creating necessary boundaries to protect the unique and innate qualities within you? Now is the time to evaluate the WHO you have become. I don't care about your achievements, the trophies in your glass case, or the accomplishments on your wall, but I do care about the self-evaluation of who you are! Take some time now to ponder these questions.

Sincerely answering these questions to yourself will help you know truly where your allegiance lies.

Have you stepped into your true power? Have you realized and magnified your passion with outstanding results because you know this exact path was created for you?

Or are you scared stiff you have become nothing more than a yes man or woman? A slave to the system and society? Running a program so instilled within you, there is no other way to think or operate other than data programmed inside your head from long ago?

It is so easy to fall into the trap of other beliefs and dogma designed to keep you a sheep herded by the whims of the world.

Are you living in truth? Are you living a life that coincides with your heart and soul? Have you become free of all the wretched pain you've experienced along the way?

Well, to not only know where we've been and where we're going, we must also look at where we currently are. Beginning an inner dialogue with ourselves is imperative, which I will expand on later throughout this book. All the answers you are seeking, believe it or not, are deep within you. The answers begin to flow once you can sit with yourself and discern what your heart is trying to say to you. This is a process that takes time and patience. To go through this process successfully, it is highly necessary to know oneself.

Because of my traumas, I developed an enormous ego, but an ego used for protection. I projected a self-centered man, even arrogant at times. However, if you were to dive a little deeper, you would come to the realization that I was nothing of the sort. I was a man with a huge heart who desperately needed to be seen and to be loved.

The stories and excuses I created became my reality. I kept manifesting all the negativity I experienced over and over, not knowing there was a completely different direction to steer.

I became addicted not only to my pain but kept a robust mental diary of everybody who had ever hurt me in the past, which was titled, *Unforgiven.*

I remembered these people when different situations triggered emotions that would surface and again reattach my hate and anger to them. I validated my feelings for them, making sure to drink the bitter poison, and I enjoyed it, even if it burned all the way down.

For so long, I was misdirected on how to move forward while shedding away so many negative emotions. This created an internal war that served as a catalyst that fueled the flames of mistrust, anger, and resentment I felt towards others and myself.

Fear dictated my every move. It had become my god, where I directed all my allegiance. My fear transformed into my anxiety, which did nothing but secure my future suffering. The pain from my past and present caused my darkness and depression and kept me from living.

Sound familiar?

These are the patterns we may subconsciously create that cause us to unknowingly enter the rat race. We can identify feeling like shit or unhappy or anxious, but we never quite understand the underlying factors as to why we feel that way.

You may have never truly leaned into yourself in the manner you should, yet simply accepted the fact that this is how you are. Therefore, you may see yourself as not deserving of the same love and attention you give unto others.

This is what you need to see instead.

This is not who you are. These are simply the symptoms of trauma and pain that have changed you without your knowledge. Now's the opportunity to become more aware.

You are worthy and just as deserving of having the same love and attention from those in your circle. But only when you see that you are worthy of it, and not from a victim standpoint, will you receive it.

So then I ask you, If you step in dog shit on the way into your house would you just deal with it and hope the smell will miraculously disappear? Of course not. You'd wash your shoe and probably set it outside for a bit just to make sure it doesn't stink up your house.

This example shows how we need to become more aware of what we are carrying and the energy we are dispersing around the ones we love.

Because of the negativity I always carried, I gave way to self-sabotage. Manifesting so much bad in my life, I unknowingly created situations for others to hurt or betray me so I could continuously confirm what I thought I already knew. This is known as confirmation bias.

I would set expectations way too high for others to meet, and I became more disengaged in certain aspects of my life so I could play the victim role when these endeavors didn't pan out.

There was no three-strikes-and-out rule with me, but one-and-done. No matter how innocent or massive the mistake, if you failed, you were out of my life forever, tagged with my hate.

My ego became my protector and executioner. With unforgiveness and malice on the frontlines, I created battles to fight every day out of nothing.

I made days that could've been seamless into a painstaking struggle with others or with myself.

A few years ago, I never knew or understood what a good or happy day was. I never enjoyed a sunset or sunrise that wasn't overshadowed by fear of a new day approaching or another sleepless night.

I never understood the power of thought or optimism. I only celebrated rainy, cloudy days because they mirrored what I always felt inside. I found distaste and agony with everything around me, never knowing gratitude and the abundant gifts that surrounded me for which I was too blind to see.

For too long, I carried the pain others projected on me, which I unknowingly took as a yoke upon my back. I allowed others to cast their self-hate and misunderstanding on me. Instead of having the power and knowledge to move through or away from it, I chose to believe it and incorporate it into my very own reality.

I realized this was not my truth, and I had the absolute power to create a new path, but it was up to me and only me to do so. I could no longer play the victim. No longer allow my ego to be in the driver's seat.

I had to *want* to change and *want* to heal. So, I began on the outside. I trained my body to operate at peak performance. This allowed me to redirect the energy toward my healing and vitality. I had to unlearn almost all of my beliefs and be humble and courageous enough to create what I thought only existed in stories with happy endings.

As I set out on my journey, I had to lean into a trust I had never known before, invoking a courage I had never used before. I trusted not in any one man or any one deity but in myself. Which, to me, is the equivalent of trusting in the one that created us.

I had to rid myself of the idea that restitution would be paid by those who wronged me, my pain would spontaneously leave me, and the life I always wanted would be laid out before me.

With humility now in the driver's seat, I headed out on a journey with what I knew, what I knew I didn't know, and an understanding that there was so much more for me to learn.

The release of control of every outcome was slowly learned with practice, while faith and power of manifestation began to be invoked in a way I had never known.

I am now able to look back on my journey with infinite gratitude and understanding rather than agonizing hate and confusion. But to get here, I had to go through many levels of hell along the way. Each presented an opportunity to shift and form myself to fit correctly in my life's path.

I had to be willing to sacrifice the old me and my old ways of thinking. I became more protective and aware of the energies that surrounded me regarding friends, family, and work colleagues. Nobody was immune to being a part of my journey.

It was time to give myself permission to heal, and by doing so, I gave myself the inherent power to be exalted and magnified.

My anger turned to energy. I began to channel my thoughts and emotions in continuous forward motion to help me move through mental barriers I never thought possible.

This is the fight. This is how I created not the life I dreamed but the life I deserve.

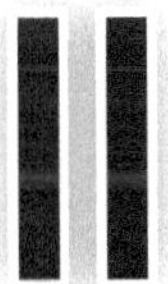

Believing in stories and confiding in your own projected limitations creates disloyalty not to the ones you hold dear but to yourself. You self-talk in a manner you never would to your kids or your partner, breaking yourself down as if you were Simon Cowell on *America's Got Talent*. Why? Because of what *you decided* to believe in so long ago.

You may have been called fat when you were younger, and even though you are not overweight, you still buy into that story. As a result, you are afraid to overeat, and you overexercise to a point where it has become unhealthy. You are subconsciously fighting an opponent that no longer exists, or perhaps never even did.

To overcome limiting self-beliefs, you must become acutely aware of your habits and be able to discern whether your behaviors are dictated by past traumas or if you are thriving and growing because of your awareness of them.

To have self-loyalty means you show up for yourself each and every day. You see the power, talents, love, and many other attributes exuded through you and for you. Finding honor and beauty in who you have become, no matter the stains or scars this life has left upon you, you continuously seek self-betterment, improvement, and to do good. You are not led by ego, nor by recognition, but you are guided by a higher power of love and virtue. Even if you do not know where your power lies precisely, you incessantly seek it.

The mere awareness of this power allows you to see yourself through a new lens. You stand firmly in you and defend your innate goodness at all costs. You do not dim your light so others feel more comfortable, nor do you apologize for the exuberant star you have become. Then you realize the side effect of allowing yourself to shine, although some may not see nor even understand. You will inspire so many to give themselves permission to step out of the program and into who they are.

You have given yourself permission to trust. You no longer ignore gut instincts and premonitions. You pay more attention to the world and signs around you.

With this work, you must be humble enough to know and trust in a greater being than yourself—a creator, an infinite supplier of goodness, power, and wisdom. With this knowledge, you shall know that this same power flows through you and for you only if you can find a way to actuate what is already there.

Trust and lean into yourself. Trust the inherent power that already exists in you. By doing so, you will see what and who can be trusted rather than being rattled around in this life like a Powerball rattles around in a cage. The narrative of hope must be switched into immediate action. You must become the creator and storyteller of your life's path and no longer defined by the limitations of your mind.

Unfortunately, self-loyalty is an entirely new concept many of us have never even conceptualized before.

To achieve self-loyalty, start by creating time to check in with yourself and your thoughts.

When you look in the mirror before you leave for the day, what is it you speak to yourself? Is it positive or hurtful? Is it encouraging or demeaning?

Can you sit with yourself in silence? Or do you always need the companionship of mood-influencing music? Do you find power in being alone? Or do you avoid it at all costs, sacrificing your time away with toxic, low-vibrational people? Do you numb yourself with alcohol or any other drugs regularly to escape your reality?

Chances are many of us have or do suffer from one or more of these things, and if you can admit it, you have grasped a power that not many can. Because, like many, we have been broken and destroyed, and I was no exception.

Over the years, we faced numerous defeats and disappointments, including heartbreaks and failures, and severe traumatic events. What we forget is that our brain does an absolutely marvelous job at recording all of those events for us, and it stores them away, so any time another similar situation comes up, it'll sound off the sirens so we can protect ourselves. Remember, the brain isn't here to make us happy; it is here to help us survive. Whenever it feels threatened, we go in flight, freeze, or fight mode. (Without getting into too many specifics of the brain and how it works, I highly recommend that you read the book *Unfuck Your Brain: Getting Over Anxiety, Depression, Anger, Freak-Outs, and Triggers,* by Faith G. Harper. It is a great reference that explains the ins and outs of severe trauma, PTSD, and how to heal from them, with a very straightforward explanation).

To move away from the pains and traumas, you must educate yourself on how to do so. And I'm sorry, prescription drugs can only aid in your journey, but there is so much more work that needs to be done from within.

I compare this to a person trying to get fit and build muscle. One needs to show up every day in the gym, do the workouts, eat correctly, get proper rest, and stick to a regimented discipline plan to see and feel their results. Then there are others who think those things are not really necessary. All they need to do is take a bunch of weight loss supplements and some protein drinks, and they will still achieve the same results, but they end up terribly disappointed.

You cannot depend on one element to find the results of healing power alone. If you go into this work, you need to do all that is necessary to be free of that which you carry.

For me, I had to dive much deeper to find out what was impeding me from moving forward. Through my self-education, I learned to call out my intention to cement it. I wanted to heal, and I wanted this monkey off my back once and for all, which was much easier said than done. But I knew that setting my intention was the crucial first step on my path to improvement.

The next step is research and discovery, or identification. Although I knew—or at least I thought I knew—everything that was holding me back, I was aware of all the traumas and heartaches I had experienced, my failures as well as my mindset. But that wasn't enough. I had to literally feel into those experiences and take myself back to each and every one of them, and then compare them to my skills and actions of the present day. Why was I always triggered in the same manner? Where did my triggers take root? How could I avoid a downward spiral that could last days or even weeks? The answers to these questions were all tethered to my past experiences.

What we need to know and remember is though talk therapy helps us in many ways, trauma is stored in the body, not just the mind. Meaning, every traumatic event that we encounter is also stored in our very organs and nervous system. (*Body Keeps Score, Kolk*, 2014). In other words, not only did I have to verbalize and talk through my traumas, I had to feel into them as well. In a way, I had to reverse engineer my current mental and emotional state.

This unforgiving man had to begin to forgive himself and others and let go of old stories. The man quick to fire from anger and blame was renovated in a manner to first search for understanding rather than immediate recoil. I had to step into courage and fearlessness to venture into the beginning, into the unknown.

I began to keep myself accountable for every action and reaction.

Was what happened in that very instance from my past still haunting me to the present day? What thought patterns occurred during each of those experiences? What painful residue was I projecting onto those around me?

It was interesting but very tough to go through each and every one of those experiences all over again. In doing so, I created a blueprint to analyze and take stock of my life leading up to now. Unfortunately, this is where a lot of people get tripped up. The thought of revisiting hidden skeletons is absolutely terrifying and out of the question, and there are those of you who have experienced things so traumatic, it looks like my life story is a walk in the park. I do know to move forward, one needs to find a way to clear out the mind and heal from whatever those experiences were.

The third, and sometimes the hardest, step is taking responsibility and being accountable for your past actions. With trauma sometimes comes an ego. Not necessarily an ego of narcissism but of protection, which is precisely what I created. As time goes by, some of us do a lot better job of falling into the victim role rather than the I-fucked-up part. We neglect the areas of our past where we were indeed responsible for whichever shitty outcome we received as a consequence for our actions. Playing the victim game in every single situation of our lives is exhausting and the foremost crippler of forward progress. Self-accountability is a power all on its own. You no longer are the victim and become the victor. It is taking the shift in focus and perspective for your experiences and putting them to bed with a productive attitude. Again, this part is for where you really fucked up. Obviously not for all circumstances.

The fourth step is forgiving yourself. Forgive yourself from whatever shame, guilt, or accountability you feel. I will dive more into guilt and shame later in this book.

Last, give yourself permission to heal. This one is trivial, and let me explain why. Self-healing gets jumbled up with all these glorifying and beautiful words that trick you into thinking it'll be a weekend in the spa, massaging out some old trigger points. But in reality, this will be the most challenging work you will ever undertake.

I am not here to sell you on your path to healing, and I am not going to make it out to be something it absolutely isn't. The work is dirty, long, messy, and even mundane at times, but the knowledge and power you gain are unparalleled, and with these few starting steps is precisely where you begin to regain self-loyalty.

These are not the steps that were given to me from a therapist or even a mentor, but what I discovered for myself. They do not need to be in that order, but this is simply what worked for me.

Throughout this book, I will discuss the power of being alone and the impactful healing attributes one gains from solitude. This is exactly how I took on this work: in complete solitude. I did everything I could to run from it, to cling to others to bear my burden for me, but to no avail. I had to take the path of *Warriorship*. So, I found other ways to self-soothe without going down a dark hole that would prove more damaging than progressive.

At the beginning of my journey, a close personal friend reached out to share a practice with me. At this point, I was open to anything, so I agreed. It was a meditative practice where I used the already identified starting mark of my trauma, which was the abandonment from my biological mother. In this meditative state, I went back to that very time when I was a baby. I envisioned myself all alone but also holding that baby as the man I was today. Tears poured out of my eyes. Initially, I felt guilty, and I was so ashamed of what the baby had gone through and was about to go through in his lifetime. Then the tears of shame became tears of fortitude. Because even before then, I realized this difficult path to healing would lead to the greatest empowerment I ever held. As I consoled my infant self, I then knew it was going to be ok, I was going to be ok, and all this shit I was undertaking would soon reveal its grand purpose; I just was not able to see it at the moment.

What we experience and the burdens we are given in this life cannot always be explained. We sometimes become so obsessed with the reason we never allow ourselves to move into healing. We search endlessly for explanations that we may never receive.

This journey does not always work out like a math equation. And to be honest, not making sense of everything happens more times than not. Our ego does a magnificent job of telling us we need to know the ins and outs of every terrible situation we face. We are programmed to think we can find peace through retribution and blame, casting the weight of the entire ordeal on someone or something else. Immediately move away from this mode of thinking. Even if the finger is pointed at ourselves, the situation is still the same. Save your time and save your energy and expend it on the path you are now creating.

Become audacious with your intentions and with your actions. Create space for what you truly seek and begin the work to authentically manifest your greatest desires. It is not only OK to explore the reasons why you love yourself, but it is also absolutely imperative you do so. It is time to be done with the negative self-talk we are accustomed to. We cling to it like flies to shit because that's precisely what it is.

In what way does negative self-talk make us better? Usually, the first response I hear from my clients is that it keeps them humble or motivated. So how often do you negatively talk to your children or your teammates or those you love most in order to motivate them? Chances are you never do. If you say all the time, then you're just an asshole, and this isn't the book for you! If your response is, "that's how I get better," you are getting that confused with constructive criticism. We all need to look at ourselves objectively and offer honest critiques to improve whatever we are working on, but it doesn't at all mean we need to be assholes to ourselves. Guess what? You can still be kind to yourself *and* be a badass at achieving the things you want most.

It is time to show up for yourself in a manner you never have before! The same way you show up for those that you love so much. You must first master the power of self-love and self-loyalty before you can truly love and be loyal to others!

It is time to begin the most crucial practice: self-love and appreciation. All of your traumas, heartbreaks, and failures may not have been completely your doing. But guess what? Getting up and healing from them is 1000 percent your responsibility and duty! It takes a conscious decision to do so. Every fucking day!

We get hung up on the most negative patterns we have fallen into. And like a magnet, we are pulled right back to them. We try so hard to cling onto faith and hope that we will soon attain whatever it is we are so desperately searching for, but our grip only lasts a few days, a few weeks, or if we're lucky, several months. Then BAM! Disappointment hits. We are let down, we are hurt, and then away we go, repeating the downward spiral into self-defeat and victim indulgence. Our old way of thinking "this is the way it is" or "no matter how hard I try, things will always be the same" creates a chasm from our progress, and we become stagnant. During times like these, we must remember we manifest what we think.

We must remember our goal to leave the old patterns of our lives, the ones that are keeping us unhappy, unfulfilled, and limiting us to what we truly deserve. We must create new patterns that are positively charged. As Rocky Balboa said in *Creed Two*, "If you want to change things in a big way, then you have to make some big changes!"

If we want to create something better, we must be loyal to ourselves, and if we don't have self-loyalty, we must find a way to create it. We will no longer sway to the ideas and opinions of others. We will no longer fall into emotional paralysis when devastation pays us for a visit. And we will no longer follow when we know we were meant to lead. Loyalty is the absolute love and power we have for ourselves. It is by self-discovery and willingness to do the work when our self-love grows and our power becomes apparent.

Create a new space allowing your self-love to grow in a way you have never thought of before. Change the narrative of "I am not worthy enough, good enough, lucky enough" to the verbal and mental affirmations of "I am worthy, and I am deserving." Say it aloud with conviction. You will amaze yourself how quickly your way of thinking and actions begin to change into good habits.

We suffer because of what we decide to believe in. So if you have done such an excellent job at manifesting the negative and pain in your life, don't you think you can just as quickly manifest the antithesis if you simply realign your focus to the positive? Think about that for a minute!

I was known as Mr. Pessimistic for a very long time for the sole reason of how I chose to believe, but I was ignorant of how to live optimistically. I thought this is just the way I was, so I accepted it to the point of self-destruction. Again, the work of healing yourself is not so simple to go and do. For many of us, our destructive behavior is like throwing a semi-truck in reverse down a highway, and so be it! Change begins with your intention and the consistency of your actions. This is the grand opportunity for you to get out of your own way. When did your negative thinking patterns ever serve you with positive results?

What about the other side of loyalty? To be loyal to ourselves, we must recognize how the damaging patterns we commit bring us down before we can ever rise. Be humble enough to know which habits you need to be rid of; this takes quite a bit of honesty and self-examination. You may already be aware of what habits you need to kick, but your consistent justification of your habits has made way for your acceptance of them, settling you into a state of being too lazy to change.

Then there is the blind loyalty we have for our friends, family, and loved ones. We feel loyalty to those we love and uphold. We think it is our duty, and with that comes a sense of honor. But what about when it comes to questioning our own integrity? Are we then being loyal to ourselves? If our personal integrity and honor come into question because of loyalty to another, the answer is most definitely no.

So you call yourself a ride-or-die friend, family member, and partner. Good for you! But standing by someone and enabling them in their ways rather than checking them in their decision making is disloyalty to yourself and whomever you've declared your loyalty to.

What if continuing to be their enabler makes us their scapegoat? We hope they'll figure it out soon. When in all reality, this reasoning is debilitating for both parties. You are obviously not helping them. By knowing better and withholding your truth, you are hurting yourself for not honoring the full circle of loyalty.

Become brave enough to create boundaries for yourself. Be ever so protective of your energies, as well as your environments. Become conscious and aware of your social circles and how these people raise or lower your vibrations.

Stop excusing yourself and those around you that may inhibit the growth and forward progress you are looking to attain.

This work can be difficult at times, but do not allow it to be deterred by excusing those around you.

If you are to be loyal to yourself and those you love, you must keep correct alignment with *all* working relationships moving forward. To do so, you must be loyal to yourself before you can be genuinely loyal to others.

It is time to show up for yourself! Ask the hard questions that you have never asked before. Lean into your past and view your life through a different lens. Shake off what no longer serves you and have the courage to walk away from the habits and people who are not in line with your direction.

Become loyal in your intentions and loyal to your heart. Become courageous in stepping into the life you know was divinely created for you. The stories and fears you created in your head are usually much more heightened in consequence than what really, if anything, plays out at all.

Being suffocated by living a life which isn't yours can quickly turn into asphyxiation.

Remove yourself from any notion that what you are about to take on needs to be easy and comfortable. Growth and change are never either of the two.

Then allow yourself to remove the label of "scary" attached to your new set path. Scary is a horror film or rushing to the bathroom at a restaurant because something didn't sit right, and you're not sure if you are going to make it on time. That's scary!

We need to reframe this work solely for what it is—work. Any negative connotation you place on it will only complicate your outlook on an already complicated situation. And as you begin to empower yourself with these divine attributes, you will no longer feel the need or desire to compare yourself to others. For you will have beauty and peace with yourself that no external factor can give you. You will become more confident in your path, with a strong and humble understanding of your life's purpose.

We can no longer be loyal to the idea that if all of the external factors in our life improve first, we will improve our attitude and life experience. Instead, we must change within ourselves before anything great can change in the outside world.

Self-loyalty, love, and trust will not be something new you are injecting into your body like a vaccine. Those qualities can be found deep within your soul, waiting to be realized and released through you.

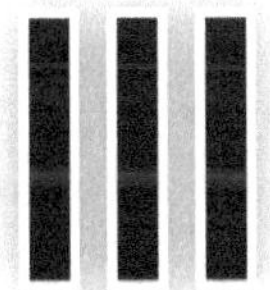

"History, despite its wrenching pain, cannot be unlived,
but if faced with courage, need not be lived again."
Maya Angelou

In 2017, I created what I felt was a fantastic health and fitness tool. We launched it on a popular crowdfunding site, and we were funded halfway through the campaign. I couldn't be more excited! Finally, I was to be launched forward in the startup world for something I created all by myself. It almost seemed too good to be true, and I would soon find out it was.

Soon after the campaign ended, my partner, who happened to be my investor, told me he could no longer be part of the project because of personal reasons. He then told me he would be pulling all the money that we raised out of the campaign to pay himself back and pay the debt we accrued along the way. He assured me not to worry because he had a big business deal coming through and would soon finance the entire project. However, his deal did not come through, but he assured me he would find me another investor who would get us there.

Because he was a trusted friend, I didn't question him. I just thought it would stretch out our timeline further.

Weeks turned into months, and months turned into two years. Although I was depending on him, I still was being proactive by setting up meetings across the country with other potential investors. Spending what little money I had to go to these meetings, he never attended one.

I desperately needed him there with me because his strength was communicating with investors; it was what he did for so many years. Instead, I was constantly given excuses for his absence.

It didn't take me long to realize he never had any intention of fulfilling his commitment.

So what was I to do? I was hopeful and felt confident I would find a saving grace to put this nightmare to an end. However, my story just sounded worse and worse to potential investors the more time went by.

I had put up everything I had for this project, and this guy literally just stood by and allowed me to be consumed by a burning inferno.

Although time passes, the wound is still in the process of healing. I began paying back investors with my own money one by one, with the minimal income I had at the time. For the first time in my life, my honor and integrity were in question.

I'm sure there are many out there who have the knowledge of how this project could've been saved. I didn't. It would've been like me handing you a rugby ball on the sidelines of the field at your first game and telling you to go sub in. Chances are you would've been scared shitless and told me no, and that's how I felt. I went from having a delegated team around me to a one-man show because the money had stopped the funding for the team.

All this transpired only a few months after I had entered into my healing journey, and like becoming sober from an addiction like alcohol, I fell into a relapse of darkness and confusion. Falling along your journey doesn't mean that the fight is over. It simply means we get to begin again and again and again until the outcome finally matches the desire of our hearts. We remind ourselves of our why, our intention, and keep going.

For me, what hurt the most were the emails I received about the project from upset backers. Because they did not know the reality of the situation, they had every right to be angry.

I am sure many of you are saying in your head, why didn't I just sell my partner out to the backers? Would that have changed my situation? Would that make all the money he took magically reappear? No, my story was the same.

Was I angry? Absolutely! This was by far the greatest betrayal I have ever experienced. I put my trust in a friend for the first time in years, and this is what I received. Perfect timing with my new acclaimed journey to self-betterment, right?

My partner would introduce me to everybody as his brother. Our bond was thicker than blood, and I thought this bond, this promise, was unbreakable. In reality, it never was even a bond, let alone a commitment. It was all one-sided.

As I reflect, I now know my hope and trust was naively misplaced. I needed this company to work so desperately, I placed too much trust not only in my partner but the team I set up around me. I went in with rose-colored glasses I don't even recall putting on.

During this time, I was nowhere near understanding the law of trust because I had not yet trusted myself. I still needed validation by others and by external factors.

Imagine the damage to my personal growth if everything would have gone according to plan. I would have validated myself based on the success of my business and not by the pure love for myself. I would have continued on the ever-failing road paved with "others' trust" rather than my own.

Then look at another perspective. What if I had completed this process of healing long before I undertook this project? Chances are desperation, and fear would have been replaced with confidence and perseverance to see it through rather than slowly fail.

The sting is still there, and I know it will eventually pass, but the invaluable lesson will be forever present. As in all things in life, there is balance in all lessons. What is shown to be good or bad will always show the opposite if you are willing to look into the situation deep enough.

Scenarios where we have to earn our pathway to healing will come alive to many of us who are wanting to take on this work. We must show up for ourselves no matter what is thrown at us. Once we start a path to healing, we sometimes fall into the trap of creating a story: All obstacles will be removed, and pure clarity will be bestowed upon us. In fact, this idea could not be further from the truth. Please do not allow that to deter you from your purpose. Instead, take a different stance than what you would have taken before you began your new journey on your new path. See the internal lessons that must be learned and incorporated within you. These are opportunities, no matter how painful they are, to make you see what was once blind to you before.

Holding malice and contempt for individuals and situations of betrayal are a hindrance we put upon ourselves. We willingly choose to carry a weight so heavy, it will debilitate every move we make toward our progress.

It is impossible to grasp on a vine and swing upward to a branch of spiritual enlightenment if we refuse to let go of the vine. We will be left in limbo, with no momentum, unless we are willing to let go and move forward.

Fixating and obsessing over *what was* does not leave space for *what is* and *what could possibly be.*

Every tough situation we endure is shitty and frightening. Especially when we have lost everything. Your power comes from deciding how to look and deal with the situation, not by becoming a slave to it.

Panic and fear are usually the resulting factors when we get thrown on our asses, and in the midst of chaos, irrational decision making often becomes imminent. Reacting out of emotion rather than logic spirals us further down than we need to go.

There is a term football quarterbacks use when they have a bad play, throw an interception, or take a few sacks called "quick memory." His job as the quarterback is not to allow those bad plays to interrupt him from being the playmaker he needs to be. Quick memory allows the quarterback to be successful by having a sound, unbreakable mindset.

If one does not have the mindset of a quick memory, they will enter into quicksand, where they are no longer in flow due to one bad play. They throw another interception, take another sack, and their performance continues to sink deeper and deeper. Like being stuck in quicksand.

Sound familiar?

We get smacked on our ass, and before we can get back up, we're hit right back down again for good measure. It is here where we are shown our strengths and weakness. We are shown exactly where we stand in the world as we know it. And like a giant universal mirror, we see exactly who we are.

It is here where we may hide in pain amid our grief. We become paralyzed in the frightening darkness. And we become dictated and run on nothing more than fear and neurotic emotions.

This is one of the scariest places to ever be. We may try and temper away the pain with distractions of work, the gym, or other hobbies we enjoy. Usually, after those have run their course through the day, we may turn to drugs and alcohol for a final escape, only to wake up the following day hungover and feeling the very same emotions as the day before. This is known as relapse. We find ourselves right back to where we were before we started this journey.

But to those who would like to take their first steps away from the darkness and confusion currently consuming them, who have had enough of the pain, weariness, and despair, I am going to tell you something you may find absolutely contrary to popular belief. USE THE DARKNESS, but do not let it use you! If you change your perspective to see yourself not as a victim of your past but as a warrior who transformed life's lessons into wisdom, then you are no longer among the downtrodden and are the master of your journey. A leader, a Warrior.

Until I started this journey, I let all my rage, fire, and anger burn deep inside me with a fucking chip on my shoulder the size of a Mack truck. I did my best to prove anybody and everybody who disrespected me, bullied me, betrayed, or hurt me wrong. The only downfall about this is although I excelled in some areas, I unfortunately failed significantly in many others.

Why?

Because I allowed the darkness to use me. I let my anger and rage dictate my every decision. Like a loose firehose at times, I was reckless and unforgiving, and I let my ego be at the forefront of my every action, but honestly, who could blame me? Who could blame you? At such a young age, I was thrown into a downward trajectory until I was able to identify and begin to work through my issues.

So, it is fair to say from birth, I was completely derailed from my true self and cast directly into confusion and distrust. My story of pain, heartache, and confusion would lead me to become the man I am today. Because I chose a new perspective and decided to go all in, my choice allowed me to create a completely different way of thinking than I ever had before.

It wasn't an easy change to become what I so much honor and love today—myself. It was a painstakingly hard process to commit to.

I like to quote Gandalf from *Lord of the Rings: The Two Towers*. When asked where he'd been, he replies passionately, "Through fire!" There's no better way for me to describe what my process was. There were days that I ultimately thought my heart was going to stop from my pain and anxiety. When I was curled up in a ball crying on the floor in devastation, accompanied by the ever-present fantasy of suicide.

I had to come to the harsh realization that healing from depression and agonizing emotional pain is not pretty or glamorous. Going back and digging into the darkest parts of your life to find some sort of reconciliation with yourself, as well as each situation, is tough.

I knew I needed to shift my self-perception from the defeated victim, with no chance of change or growth to a warrior who says, "I fucking got this!"

Because I had convinced myself I was a mistake, it was difficult for me to make this transition. My mother obviously didn't want me, neither did this sideways society I grew up in, and though I had hard evidence to support my feelings, it still didn't improve my way of living one damn bit! Instead, it stunted any potential growth I desperately needed.

For a few years after my startup went under, I couldn't get hired or even interviewed. I felt as though the very floor beneath my feet was crumbling away. Panic was at an all-time high, and my anxiety was through the roof. All because I was running on a program that was not my own. I had become a follower of other paths rather than the creator of my own.

So instead of empowering myself, I was consistently giving my power away.

I thought of all the things I would be willing to do to relieve myself of this torment or to just start with a clean slate, with no recollection of the burdens I had been carrying. Rescued away from my pain and sorrows was an everyday fantasy.

We are not wrong to think this way. We are not wrong to feel confused or angry as to why we do not experience happiness and success as we believe others around us do. Where we do fail time and time again is believing that there is nothing we can do to change and correct our course.

If we can shift our focus to inside of ourselves and away from all the distractions then we can see where to begin the work. It took me many years of testing and trying different methods that worked best for me to see and incorporate change. Before then, I lived out the toxic clichés of "if you don't love me at my worst, you don't deserve me at my best" or "take me as I am."

I felt I had earned the right to be an asshole to myself and those around me. My ego had gone into hyperdrive, and the facade of not caring and self-preservation was all a show.

I realized my ego did a phenomenal job lying to me and making me believe my weakest and most negative attributes were my strongest. I was fooled into thinking all should respect me because of my past, and I should be forgiven easier for my misdeeds and shortcomings. Never once seeing that my own toxicity was a burden I was passing on to my surroundings.

We are even excused by people saying, "Don't mind them; they've had a hard life." As if my story had warranted me acting careless and insensitive to others.

For too long, I felt justified in my anger, carrying a cloud of dark energy with me wherever I went. As I now look back, I feel embarrassment for the burden I cast upon those around me, especially those whom I genuinely care for.

As I recognized and took power in my growth, I realized it was deep inside me: the hurt, abused, let down, abandoned, inner child who had been greatly affected by my ability to move forward.

The man I had grown into created a desire to be more social, more interactive with others, but I was continuously brought back to the place of fear and distrust. Fear that others wouldn't like the real me, and distrust for if they did, in some way, they'd find a way to betray me. So here I was, stuck in quicksand, so desperate to move forward, but paralyzed by the inability to do so.

In the book *12 Rules for Life*, Jordan B. Peterson likens the human experience to lobsters because of our closely related nervous system. After a battle deciding male dominance, territory, and mating rights, the defeated lobster's brain is dissolved, and he grows a new, subordinate brain. Peterson goes on to share that if the subordinate lobster gathers enough courage to fight again, he is statistically likely to lose again.

For a man who was used to winning at sports his whole life, I began to lose, over and over again, and I questioned my every move with insecurity leading my way. My unhealed traumas of childhood had greatly impeded my adulthood. Fears, lies, and the stories I created became my waking reality. I was like a defeated lobster. Although willing to fight again, I only continued to lose. At this point, I manifested my failures because I expected to lose.

Defeat is devastating for anybody in sports, business, relationships. Some of us can learn immediately from our misfortunes and bounce back better and stronger, but I couldn't. I snowballed to the bottom of the hill, and no matter how much I tried to make my way to the top, I was ice skating uphill.

So, how did I change my victim mentality? How did I change my trajectory entirely and gain momentum in the right direction after so many losses?

I had to lean into trust. For the first time in my life, I had to wholeheartedly learn something I thought I was incapable of knowing.

What is so tricky about trust is that if it was taken, broken, or betrayed, that feeling is forever ingrained within you. Those memories of trauma, fear, abandonment, and abuse stay relevant to the point of coating your DNA. And unless you've taken the proper measures to heal, these genes can easily be passed down to your children (Kellermann, 2011).

According to (Kellermann, 2011), epigenetics is typically defined as the study of heritable changes in gene expression that are not due to changes in the underlying DNA sequence. Such heritable changes in gene expression often occur as a result of environmental stress or major emotional trauma and would then leave certain marks on the chemical coating, or methylation, of the chromosomes (Meaney & Szyf, 2005). The coating becomes a sort of "memory" of the cell, and since all cells in our body carry this kind of memory, it becomes a constant physical reminder of past events—our own and those of our parents, grandparents, and beyond. "The body keeps the score" (van der Kolk, 1994), not only in the first generation of trauma survivors but possibly also in subsequent ones. Because of their neurobiological susceptibility to stress, children of Holocaust survivors may thus easily imagine the physical suffering of their parents and almost *remember* the hunger, the frozen limbs, the smell of burned bodies, and the sounds that made them scared. This kind of epigenetic cell memory can possibly explain how elements of experience may be carried across generations, as described by Perry (1999).

Although epigenetic therapy is somewhat new, there are many treatments available when professionally diagnosed.

So here comes your responsibility once again: If you know for a fact you come from a line of slavery, holocaust, war, etc., it is your responsibility to heal. What a great opportunity you have been given! You now get to not only heal yourself but the generations that came before you. Now before you go running scared, hang with me. This isn't scary work; this is what you are made of. This is what you and only you can do, and that excites me, and it should excite you as well. I'm not going to use the time now to explain how epigenetic therapy works; look it up if your heart calls you to. It's phenomenal work.

So how do you find trust when trust itself was never learned? How do you find self-love when you were never loved? First, by simply setting an intention to do so. Sounds easy, right? So let's think about this.

Every night before you go to bed, most likely you set a few intentions for the next day, correct? Also known as the checklist for tomorrow: vacuum the house, mow the lawn, take the kids to practice, or get dog food. Each day you will most likely accomplish these simple intentions with action, but these actions are not rewiring my brain to think in a way I never felt before, right!?

One of the most important things I can tell you when it comes to healing and setting something as easy as an intention is don't overcomplicate an already complicated situation. If you look back on your life, there are hundreds of things you learned to do that you never thought you'd be able to, simply because you first set an intention then put that intention into practice.

Here is a very easy mantra to think of and apply in your own life. TRUST IN YOUR TRUST AND NOT IN YOUR FEAR.

To be able to learn trust, you must begin to make space for it. To do that, you must filter your mind of mistrust. So how do you do that? By clearing away fear as soon as it enters your conscious mind.

As humans, many of us fester in our fears longer than we play in our greatest desires, which is why so many of us suffer from mental illness, anxiety, and depression. We have to take over our mind with constant repetition and practice just like we learned new trades and abilities we once doubted we could ever learn. We must not only train our mind but completely retrain and rewire the stories we once thought were true.

Immediately identify when the negative thoughts enter and refocus on the positive or something other than the negative. It all starts with an intention, then the consistent follow-through of action each and every day.

Imagine for a minute, and soon as often as you can, a life where you no longer feel the need to explain yourself to others. Imagine simply walking into a room not caring so much about what others may think of you or how they may be judging you. This concept is not removed from reality but very much an attainable goal. This power comes from within, never from external validation or assuredness.

We may think the money and extravagant lifestyles we see on social media correlate to self-love and real confidence. That is a lie so many of us buy into. We know those people seem to have everything, but we also know some of them personally, who deep down are not happy, and they may not even know why. Perhaps because they are also human and experience the same kind of situations we all do, they just have more glitter and glitz.

There will always be a "they." Those whom we are continually comparing ourselves to or wishing we could be like. Again, thinking like this is creating unnecessary obstacles that do not need to be in our path. No matter which story we choose to believe, to hold onto the power of trust and self-love, one must do the work from the inside out to truly obtain it.

I began to finally find my power when I fully accepted my story. I was able to see the truth that was there and recognize the lens and masks I wore that prohibited me from being my best self. I no longer turn my face to what has happened and run away, desperately hoping to lose them.

Trust was devastatingly hard for me to understand, therefore a great challenge to create in my own life. It seemed like every time I trusted or was trusted, it was destroyed in blistering fashion.

I was giving away the illusion of trust, but in reality, I never had any real trust to give. I was living a life on borrowed credit and overspending much more than I earned where trust was concerned.

This is how we topple and blame our situations on the world. We leave no room for accountability or self-realization, for that which we continue to manifest is that which we continue to believe.

This path is measured by level upon level and layer upon layer. If the lesson is not learned, the same obstacle will linger or return differently, time and time again.

Now, rather than allow my circumstances to enrage me, I do give myself permission to be upset and even angry, but I also allow these emotions to pass, so I will make more logical pragmatic decisions thereafter. I now realize the power I have to take over myself.

There is always an opportunity to react out of the past. Sometimes our reactions are charged with old pain and triggering memories. But when you step in the realm of consciousness, those excuses become quickly outdated.

There may not always be an answer or an explanation for everything we have gone through, but there can always be a lesson if we are willing to lean in deep enough to find it.

Remove yourself from the darkness and confusion. Allow pain and rage to come but no longer dictate your every emotion. Use the darkness by allowing yourself to take the lessons into newly found wisdom and resolve.

You are no longer the victim of your story. Take up arms, turn and fight your way back to who you are destined to be!

IV

"To be free from all suffering, free yourself from attachment."
Buddha

Many of us have heard miraculous stories about couples trying to get pregnant. They spend thousands of dollars on different medications and procedures. Their sex life turns into a work hour, but unfortunately for some, their miracle of pregnancy never comes true. After investing tons of money and time with no return on success, they hang it up. These results can be devastating for the couple, but for some lucky others willing to push through, they begin to let go of hope and start looking to alternative means of adding to their family.

Stress and worry leave, and they completely let themselves go of any expectation. It's then the baby is conceived. The reason I'm sharing this is to tell you that attaching yourself to the outcome of any situation can be devastating if it doesn't work out as you anticipated.

Now don't get what I'm saying confused with settling for something less than what you feel you deserve; that's not at all what I'm trying to explain.

Let me share another example to better illustrate what I'm trying to convey.

My good friend in Los Angeles is a very successful actor. When I accompanied him to an audition, I asked if he stresses over being hired for the gig. He said, "I practice and train, perfecting my craft every day. I do my best at each audition then I never think about it again. If I get the part, awesome! If not, I know there will always be other auditions, no point in worrying about them, it's simply a waste of time." He had figured out the process. Do everything you can in your power to achieve the best possible outcome, but don't be emotionally attached to the end result.

In 2000, I signed my scholarship to play college football. I knew I was on my way. I just needed two or three good years, then I'd fulfill my dream of playing professionally on Sundays. Not for the fame, and not even really for the money, but because I absolutely loved the game of football. That dream literally came to a crashing end when I was t-boned in an intersection at 80 miles an hour. Game over.

I didn't have a plan B. I was not just a player but a student of the game of football, and before I knew it, it was all gone.

I became lost, confused, and even angrier than before. How did this happen? I was told if I worked hard, harder than anyone else, my dream of running down the sideline would come true. That's the belief we buy into. For some, it may work out as hoped, but not for me.

I had become so attached to the outcome that when it was gone, devastation and despair grew deep within me. I started making irrational decisions as I tried to pick up the pieces and start my life over. I allowed the world to tell me what decisions I should make, from the kind of job I should pursue to whom I should choose for a relationship. Before I knew it, my path to darkness and rage had widened before me, and down the rabbit hole, I went.

Because I was attached to one possible outcome, when the opportunity to pursue that outcome was taken away, my identity went with it. I defined who I was by what I did. It's not necessarily the loss of hope that devastates us but the failed expectation. We as humans become so emotionally connected to our expectations that each specific outcome makes us either happy or sad, disappointed, or relieved. We limit ourselves to view the world in black or white, never seeing the beauty of all the colors around us.

Here is another simple example. Just to make sure we're still following along.

Say we have a date with our significant other, and it's been such a long time since we have gotten to spend quality time together. So we have a plan. Dinner reservations at 7 p.m. at your favorite restaurant, then go to a movie at 9 p.m. This gives us just enough time to get back to the babysitter and enjoy a dedicated evening with each other.

Your wife calls at 6:30 p.m. and says she is running late because she got held up at work. You're annoyed because you're expected at the restaurant in 30 minutes. She arrives just at 7 p.m., and she knows you're upset because of the missed reservation. You begrudgingly decide to eat at another restaurant that does not require reservations and spend the entire night not speaking to each other because the evening didn't follow your original plan. You both decide to go back home, although you could've still seen the movie. Night wasted! All because expectations were not met. Rather than being grateful for a night together without the kids and finally having some "us" time, you are both annoyed with each other.

Now how often do we let little experiences like this go to waste because of the most insignificant of circumstances? Sometimes we need to take a step back and look at the bigger picture.

Of course, there are deadlines that need to be met and deals that need to be closed so we can make quota. But every time something doesn't go the way we imagined, sadness, disappointment, and even depression follow.

The experiences in our lives aren't meant to be always in accord with our desires. Growth is predicated upon adversity, let downs, and failures, but only if we choose to learn from whatever lesson is being taught.

We are not often motivated to ask, *"Hmmm, what can I learn from this?"* It is more likely after the dawn has passed and the sun has risen we can reflect on what exactly was gained.

Did I move upward spiritually? Did I grow wiser from my mistakes? Or did I become harsher and guarded from a broken heart?

With every action is an opposite and equal reaction, according to Newton's third law of motion. With that law, we are all given a choice on how to react no matter the situation. We do have that power.

Just like any craft, this power to control our reactions takes time to develop and practice. Most of us have, unfortunately, lived through horrific events that have forever changed us. But as I mentioned in the previous chapter, it is imperative to ask yourself if these events have used you and defined you. Or have you used these events and defined them? That's the bridge I am trying to connect!

For so long, my trauma used me in every decision I made, and because of it, I was incessantly attached to every waking outcome. I was so desperately depending on these events to make me happy, to change the course of my angry, confused life. I believed every time I would end up disappointed, and every time I was. I needed just one of the magical fantasized events to change my course, so I would pray and hope they would come into fruition, but they never did.

Why?

I was a good person, at least in my eyes. Why couldn't God hear me? Or even see me? Everyone around me seemed like they were living their best life. When was it my turn to have my seat at the table? To be seen? To be recognized?

The one and ultimate lesson I had to learn, what I was drastically searching for externally, was what I needed to search for internally. I finally did. No more external validation, no more desperate pleas for things to work out perfectly how I wanted. It was time to find who I inherently was. It was time to let go of all control and ALLOW the universe to do its job. So what is within us that makes us feel we need to be in control of every situation? Ask yourself. Chances are it will always come right back down to ego and fear. Fear of not having control of the outcome, and ego for not having control of the situation. This is how they are connected. Fear empowers the ego just as the ego empowers fear. To make a place of allowance, we must first leave the ego behind and step into a place of faith in and patience for the process.

We can no longer make irrational decisions based on traumas, victimization, and hopelessness. Do not allow yourself to be disillusioned by your pain greeted with irrationality. Instead, welcome awareness and courage.

Einstein once said, "Imagination is more important than knowledge. Knowledge is limited, imagination encircles the world. Logic will get you from A to B, but imagination will take you anywhere." Having things always work out the way you want isn't necessarily always beneficial, even though your way seems easier and more gratifying. There is no growth or forward movement created from a perfectly easy path.

For so long, I was ingrained with negativity and pessimism. I always imagined the worst, and the worst was always manifested. Just as I had the power to create my physical body to perform the way I intended it to, I had to learn to retrain my brain. I had to rid it of all the negativity with nothing but a constant barrage of emotional and mental explosions going off. This feat was more than challenging, and at times, I felt it was impossible. I had to take my brain and change the direction of my thought processes. To push it in a way it had never known. To no longer use my abandonments, heartbreaks, failures, rejections as vices any longer.

Not only did I need to remove attachment to any future outcomes but attachments to all my past experiences, which were viciously writing my story and current conditions present day. To consciously step away from my identity of pain altogether.

There are so many of us out there who are so afraid to leave their past behind. Afraid to do the work because they are so attached to their past traumas. Fearful of what they might find under all the scars and facades created, but this is a fight we can no longer shy away from. It is the fight and the battle we must undertake with an undaunting will and relentless perseverance.

I was once told "you can stay in your shit or do something about it." There has to be a point in your life when you are tired. Tired of the pain, tired of feeling sorry for yourself, and tired of not taking your place of power.

It's time to get out of your shit and step into your God-given power with the understanding that the direction you choose to go will not always be in your control, set with only your outcomes.

Chances are, comfort and the thought of venturing into the unknown may discourage you from taking these first steps.

You need to come to the point where you are past reading, liking, and posting motivational memes, gifs, and quotes on social media. Feeling the quick shot of dopamine to the brain is not going to give you the power to step up into yourself and do the work.

Quit faking who you are to the strangers following you. Set your phone down and do the fucking work!

Social media has fooled you into believing the amount of likes and followers you have translates into happiness and success. So many of you are willing to buy fake followers, likes, and comments to make you feel better and more credible. When in reality, you're so unhappy and lonelier than ever before because you have become so dependent on a stranger's double tap than authentic interaction with others, and more than that, with yourself.

I also fell into the trap. I spent hundreds of dollars building a decent following simply because I wanted to look credible, but I realized the pure hypocrisy I was living. I was talking and speaking truths to others and doing everything to live it myself, but I was a lie on social media. After about a year hiatus from social media entirely, I brought it back and deleted every fake follower there was. My following was cut by nearly 80 percent. I know many Instagram gurus would say that was foolish, but for me to live in truth, I must be truthful in all facets of life.

It seems this generation has glamorized the single party life—it has become an outright deceiver of the quality of life—and become lost, believing the quantity of followers equates to the blissfulness of existence rather than the quality of truth.

We have tricked our brains into thinking the more significant the influencer, the happier one must be. How can I up my following? Why isn't my content being validated? Why does nobody like me? That's the beginning of a very dangerous spiral. There are many times where I caught myself and realized I was searching to fill a very shallow bucket of self-esteem, validated by thousands of people whom I don't even know. People that have no idea of my story, nor will ever know the path I took to get where I am today.

This is a common, dangerous trap of attachment we have become so accustomed to, and it is nothing but a lie. Your following nor your likes equate to who you are as a person! Let me repeat!

YOUR FOLLOWING NOR YOUR LIKES EQUATE TO WHO YOU ARE AS A PERSON!

The longer you continue to compare, emulate, and pretend you are someone you are not, the longer you will prolong your suffering. For you are denying the truth deep within you.

To that regard, we must look at how we are representing ourselves to the rest of the world.

Are you selling someone on social media who doesn't even exist? Are you deceiving your audience and followers with filters that do not show your true identity? Are you showing off locations, cars, and riches, that aren't yours? And if they are, what is the message you are trying to convey?

Are you posting half-naked photos because you are so desperate for attention and validation that you are literally willing to take it all off? These are examples of attachment you are seeking in a very artificial world.

This need and desire you carry to be wanted, to feel as though you belong will never be fulfilled by anything or anyone other than yourself!

I am sorry you feel loneliness. I am sorry you feel invalidated or not wanted, but the small screen on your phone will never completely fill that void. One must take to the work and find those resolutions within. Only within, can emptiness be replaced with sound fulfillment.

Allow yourself to use the advantages and entertainment of social media but take your power back to no longer allow the false promises of social media to dictate or validate who you are as a person. Find your inner greatness, strength, and power without the distraction of social media platforms or opinions of strangers that lead you to doubt the person you are becoming.

Change your viewpoint to focus on your gifts that will fulfill your potential.

We often see in our lives the challenge of becoming selfless. Putting others always before us, right? I believe that is one of the most significant lies ever told! I believe you can be selfish while putting the ego aside completely. It is time we look at the word selfish under a completely different light. Why are many of us afraid to put ourselves first before others? Are we kind to others because we know the pain from abuse all too well? Do we love so hard because we know what it is like to not be loved? Do we laugh and joke to cover up the painful reality we face? If you answer yes to any of these questions, I challenge you to take on a whole new perspective and begin to show up for yourself with consideration of selfishness.

It is time to work on you before you feel called to work on others in order to facilitate the healing process. Practice self-love, then apply self-love. Learn to love yourself for the first time in your life, without conditions or because of imperfections. Learn to love all of you with your faults. Accepting who you are entirely creates room to fall in love with the process of finding your higher self. Dismantle fear and loosen the grip of control.

"Perfect love drives out all fear." (1 John 4:18)

We can learn to move away from the desperate fear of dependent love and become centered in the power of abundant love from deep within ourselves.

This method applies to trust, kindness, and whichever divine ability you feel you need to foster in your own life. When you learn to live in trust or any of the divine abilities, you will then bestow them in the world and people around you.

Call it self-care, selfishness, or any word you feel. Realize that learning these sacred divine attributes does not inflate the ego with narcissism but will enable you to harness your power to magnify and move you into your true and higher purpose.

Show up for yourself FIRST! Rather than looking to others to vainly fulfill whichever attachment concept you lack. Then you will have the power to show up for everyone else after.

Rid yourself of attachment. Still give your all but allow yourself space not to be hurt because of desperation for your specific outcome. If you can take the time to sit with yourself over every heartbreak you've suffered, especially those where you were so attached to a specific outcome, you will be able to see the light gained from the loss.

Again, this comes with a substantial amount of awareness. If all goes according to plan, then the contrary is usually never even noticed. It is only when the negative appears do we realize the lessons if we so choose. But to disregard attachment, we must also be willing to let go of control.

To exercise restraint or direction over; to hold in check; to eliminate or prevent. These are all definitions of control we as humans egotistically love to exhibit. We are hardwired to be control freaks, usually with one or more aspects of our lives.

Do you feel the need to always be the one driving? I do! Are you the one to always do the laundry or mow the lawn? Whatever "that" is, we need to have complete control over it, but why? Because we like it done our way. Even if there are so many eligible hands to help us with the task, we still do not afford them the opportunity to do so.

To complete the entire spectrum, we must determine if our need to be in control of all aspects of our lives is a hindrance or a help to our growth.

We control what we can and detach ourselves from what we cannot. So I ask, Are you in the state of constant control? Or have you given yourself permission to accept that some things run their natural course, rather than stress over controlling what you cannot? If you strive to control everything, how is that serving you? What fears occupy every space of your subconscious and conscious thoughts so you have no room for allowance?

It is here we must revert back to the tool of identification, or research and discovery, in order to understand the narratives that lead us to believe that not only must we have control over every situation but we must also have control over every outcome.

Imagine if when you were young, you got in a terrible car accident as a passenger, which wasn't your fault, and since then, you refuse ever to let anyone else drive. In essence, it is a very valid reason. We've all experienced something and looked back and said to ourselves, "If I were in charge of it, it never would've happened!" Maybe that's true in some cases, but let's be honest, not in all.

So while you are busy doing your best to control every situation, let me guess. I am sure you are calm, collected, and at complete peace, right? Yeah, didn't think so! You may think you are in control, but you have simply given away all your power to the ego. You're fearful, worried, stressed, and anxious.

Now, if you are a complete mastermind of your craft like some of the greatest sports legends and coaches, perhaps you know exactly what to expect after every play because you have it down to a science, and you have practiced and created every scenario to make sure every play is practically foolproof. So unless you are Bill Belichick, Kobe Bryant, or Michael Phelps, or equal to them in your mindset, it's time to start putting this practice into play.

This is the art of surrender and allowance. To allow stress and anxiety to turn into peace and stillness. You are no longer fearful for the future because you have created a space to live in the present, and with this comes the power to see more than you would using narrow tunnel vision. It yields way for even more opportunities rather than being consumed by an uncertain outcome.

This is also true for our relationships. So many of us—including myself—have been attached to the outcome of conditional love. If my partner does this, then I will love her more, but if she doesn't fulfill and show up for me in this exact way, I will love her less. Because of trust issues and past pain, our relationships become dependent on the fulfillment of predetermined expectations. For many, there is no room for error. I am not talking about egregious mistakes only. I am talking about small mistakes made into significant arguments simply because a little expectation was not met, or our partner did not respond the way they were supposed to respond. We disregard what else they may be carrying from that day. We are so quick to crucify the person we love most, or ourselves, because perfection was not met.

Take a step back and reexamine how your expectations play out with your significant other. Are you so hard on them they have no room for mistakes? Or perhaps your expectations and leniency are too low, causing another sort of problem. You must create a space for alignment and growth. You are not perfect either; therefore, allow the same space for error for yourself as you would for those whom you love.

If you feel stuck in a specific situation, there may be a chance you have set yourself on one route, and therefore, only one outcome. For so long, that was my program. I could not move or be happy until the scenario played out exactly how I imagined it in my mind. It wasn't until I was able to let go of all control that I could force my path open.

Remember, surrendering and letting go of control is not letting go of power; it is standing within your power! Have the faith and patience to let things play out as they must after you have done everything possible to produce the best result.

V

"Anyone can be a father, but it takes someone special to be a dad,
and that's why I call you dad, because you are so special to me.
You taught me the game, and you taught me to play it right."
Wade Boggs

Throughout my entire athletic career, I've always had one tradition after every game, whether it is after a football or rugby game.

When we were done shaking hands with the opposing team, and after we heard Coach's final thoughts, I'd go take a shower. These showers were always particularly long. Not because I was sore or tired but because I'd get stuck in thought as I rehearsed each play in my head. Like I was watching the film on the game I played, I'd reflect on everything I did wrong no matter how well I played. If I had scored five tries in a rugby game or rushed for over 300 yards in a football game, it was never what I remembered. I only concentrated on what kept myself from perfection, and I'd replay those instances in my mind over and over. I'd muddle over what I should've and could've done differently and better. Because of this post-game ritual, some of these showers would last more than an hour until the water ran cold.

I do not consider myself a perfectionist, but I do consider myself a man that beats himself up more than most, and in retrospect, I realize this is more of a weakness than a strength. This is true in every facet of my life except one: fatherhood.

I have been divorced for more than seven years. I moved out when my daughter was only six months old. Her mother and I tried for almost five years to reconcile, but in the end, I decided I did not want my daughter living in an unhealthy household seeing her parents fight all the time. So after years of counseling, it was time to walk away.

Over and over, I kept playing the marriage in my head. Should I have suffered through this marriage for the sake of my daughter? What would I be teaching her if I did? Selfishly, there's a part of me that wanted to stay so I wouldn't miss one aspect of her life, but I knew for my own emotional and mental health, it was time to move on.

Her mother and I are still trying to figure out this thing called divorce. We have some great weeks and great months, and others not so much. Even though we're not always on the same page, I can absolutely say that she is an amazing mother.

Divorce is an interesting occurrence in life. We've been taught the person we once loved and exchanged vows with immediately turns into our mortal enemy. We've been taught to villainize our former spouse to our family and friends so they can believe our own innocence or justify any unlawful actions during our marriage and thereafter.

One thing I've come to realize is divorce sucks no matter what. And although it may be liberating and exceptionally healthy, it still has its severe growing pains and heartbreak.

We once made a commitment with all our hearts to this person, and then all of a sudden, it's over. But, guess what? We don't have to suck at being divorced. It's hard enough when kids, assets, or businesses are involved. Yes, they're times that call for complete due process. There are times when your heart has been ripped out, run over with a car, spit on, then backed over again, and we can think of nothing else more than to have that person feel the way they made you feel with complete retribution.

As our ego takes over, we sometimes forget about what is most important—the children. During this awful time, we are easily triggered, we are tired, and we are looking for nothing else but the future and for this chapter to finally be over and done with.

So it is very easy to not be mindful about how we can unknowingly pass our traumas onto the most innocent bystanders. All kids will experience some sort of stress. Some experience post-traumatic stress disorder due to a divorce. It all depends on the child and how severe the separation is between the parents. Divorce can show how powerful our energies are as parents, which can vibrate all the way to our children.

Let's then talk about all the bullshit consequences and egotistical reactions caused by divorce.

Men, I'm still amazed that I have to convey this message repeatedly.

Pay your child support!

I don't care if she isn't using the money for your child, pay it! As men, we must honor our commitments, even when they are unfair or lopsided. By doing so, you are honoring yourself and your divine purpose. Trust me, I know and understand you question the use of these funds when you know they aren't appropriately spent. Especially if your income is limited, but the essential concept is knowing your children are being taken care of. (I'll move on to the mother's responsibility shortly.)

Second, make time for your children!

Spend all the time you possibly can with them. Teach your children, lead them, guide them, but most of all, listen to them. Hear what they have to say.

Not too long ago, I was with my daughter, and we were getting treats for movie night. She picked out a chocolate bar and said, "I want this one." I quickly grabbed the bar from her hand and put it back. "Babe, you don't want this one." I then grabbed my favorite chocolate and gave it to her. "This one is the best, trust me!" I arrogantly told her. She looked at the chocolate with her head down, and we proceeded to leave the store. As we drove off, I looked in the back seat and could see she was visibly sad. "Mars, what's wrong, girl?" With her seven-year-old voice, she said, "Dad, I didn't want this chocolate, I wanted the other chocolate bar. Just because you like this one doesn't mean I can't like the other one I picked out." I slowly sunk in my seat. Dammit, she was so right! I immediately apologized and offered to go exchange it, but it was too late, and my ego had made the decision for her without honoring her as the pure, beautiful soul she was. Luckily, seven-year-old daughters are quick to forgive their fathers when they mess up. I was genuinely grateful for the lesson.

Some of us men do a great job at forcing our will upon our children, instead of having the patience to listen and hear. We forget how so many of us were rebellious to our parents.

As fathers, we need to protect our children at all costs. When they're young, we do have to make individual decisions for them, but in no way do we need to make all of them. As a father, we must be able to let go of control and let our children make decisions on their own, even at a young age. By doing so, they will build autonomy. Remember, even though they are of you, it does not mean they are you. Be humble enough to learn from your children, even at such an innocent and inexperienced age. They see things that we have simply forgotten how to see. They find joy in almost everything. Allow those aspects to come back and be a part of you once again. Do not allow this life to go by without impacting their lives as much as possible. And by doing so, they will affect yours just as much. Even if you have dishonored yourself with past decisions and you do not feel worthy of being in their presence, fight to become worthy. Worthiness is an absolutely necessary trait of a father.

Third, the old ways of teaching your children to be tough by being emotionally unavailable to them are just that, old and obsolete.

When we do this as men, we are not only shaming our children with their emotions, but we are not allowing them to truly honor how they feel. We can create trauma or emotional disconnection in our children. This may result in our children suffering from self-doubt, inner turmoil, or "daddy issues" because they hopelessly searched for your approval.

Last, tell them how much you love them!

Compliment them on qualities other than their appearance and let them see YOU! In turn, you will help them gain the confidence they need to create self-power and give themselves permission to be who they truly are. That's how fucking powerful we are as fathers, and how decimating we can be if we do not invoke this inherent power.

Now, women, mothers, queens. I am speaking to you now. Men have always gotten a bad rap for being a deadbeat dad. You rarely hear of the deadbeat mom, and there are thousands of examples to justify both sides. The one important topic that needs to be addressed and understood is if the father of your children is loving and caring, do not keep your children away from him out of spite, no matter what occurred between you two! If you have done this and continually do this, you have dishonored yourself and severely limited the positive impact, security, and potential growth of your children just so you can feed your ego. You have to realize it's not about you! It's about the children.

Allow me to clarify. There are different circumstances where mothers need to keep their children safe, but I'm speaking to those women that unlawfully keep their children away from good fathers. Change it! And get out of your own way!

Another difficult situation for me to see and even experience at times in these relationships has been the slander by one or both parents and their family in front of the children.

Doing this paints a very unfair and false image between the sanctity of the parent(s) and their children, no matter the grievance. I had always made it a point never to speak ill of my daughter's mother, and I never have. Not because there haven't been times I've wanted to, but only because it hurts nobody but my daughter.

I want my daughter to look at her mother as Wonder Woman, with purity and beauty. So let me reiterate. YOU ARE HURTING NOBODY BUT YOUR CHILDREN! If you are rationalizing to yourself why you are doing any of these things listed above, then I am specifically speaking to you!

Go vent to your best friend, your mother, your trainer, your therapist, but stop tarnishing the innocent image of what your child has created of the other parent. It only causes more confusion and heartbreak on top of what they might have already experienced with your divorce or separation.

Now, I started this chapter by explaining my post-game ritual. Dissecting everything I did wrong that kept me from perfection, and somehow, I've taken that same ritual into fatherhood. I reflect on each situation and decide if there is something I could've done better. Did I project my own stress or current life situation on my daughter by the way I reacted to a situation? Was I too hard on her and not sensitive enough? Did I say or do something that was not in line with my true self? I know I'll never be perfect, but I will do everything I can to be perfect for her, and I know I still have so far to go. Do not ever settle into "this is who I am" or "this is how I was raised." Seek to be better, seek to allow your true divine self to be uncovered and shared with those most critical and most affected by what you choose to exude.

There needs to be a time of reckoning for yourself, where you can no longer put your shitty current circumstances on your ex. I understand how harsh this may sound for those in dire states of affairs, but as I have stated before, playing the victim of your current condition does not help you. Think of what your children see and the example you are showing them as you sit in your pity. Then think of the man or woman who gets off their ass with the odds stacked against them and creates a beautiful life for themselves and their children. Imagine the resounding impact this will have on your kids! They will witness an example of invincibility and think, "If my mom can do it, I can do it!"

Your example matters more than your words ever have!

With the example you put forth comes self-examination of the very traits you are carrying and may be passing on to your children. The good and the bad. Being understanding because you were raised a certain way does not at all make it right. This includes cultural and religious traditions. We continually fall into this trap of tradition. We have learned and taught and relearned and retaught the same unhealthy customs and traits that have been passed on from generation to generation, and with those come the same traumas that were passed on again and again. Just because it was passed on and taught to you does not give you the right to allow it in your household. It is time to end that which does not serve the greater good under your roof. Take a step back and ask yourself these questions: Does it make me and mine happy? Does it build confidence within the household? Does it make everybody feel safe? Do these teachings bring shame? Do they bring fear? If you are honest with these questions, you will know which to follow and which to drop.

Be willing to have an open dialogue within your family. Search and ask for data. What may be working great for one family or family member may not necessarily be working great for yours.

We must know we are the only ones responsible for ending the vicious unhealthy cycles within our family units. It is time we stand with accountability and shoo the non-serving ideals away.

Create time to open up conversations in a safe environment among you and your family. You may be surprised what is revealed. By doing so, you will create a stronger foundation and a more peaceful refuge for all to return each day.

The entire premise of this book is to find and uphold your true and divine self. It also holds true to your family. Finding the true and divine identity of your family and stepping into the power that magnifies each other like a well-oiled machine. Do not let ego run your family unit, nor old, outdated traditions.

Now please note, there are many absolutely great traditions and customs throughout the world that strengthen a family unit. As the parent, you must decide which ones do not suit you and which ones strengthen you.

Do not force your child to fulfill your failed dreams. No matter how close you came and whichever circumstances caused them not to fall into fruition. Allow them to step into their own power; be their guide, their confidant, and primary source of wisdom, but in no means force them to do something just because it runs in the family. They will most likely find resentment and rebel in their own way.

All my life, I have seen parents push their children into the same sports and hobbies they grew up with. Waterboarding their children with practice after practice, clinic after clinic, and game after game. Parents pushing them to achieve greatness, superiority, and fame, but at what cost? I have seen children detach themselves from their parents because of the slave-driven mentality they are pushed by. I see them lose love for an activity they once enjoyed with all of their heart.

Communicate with your child to know what their true aspirations are and what kind of load they are willing to take on along with their school and other responsibilities. Do not allow a wedge of frustration and annoyance to come between you and yours because communication was not present or genuine opinion was not taken into consideration.

We need to fall out of the old programming that to have a successful family, x, y, and z all need to be checked off. Guess what? Chances are, not all your kids are going to want to go to college or even do things the exact way we did growing up. If they do, great! If not, give them the power of choice if their path isn't aligned with yours. Now I am not speaking about letting them run free like it's the 1960s all over again. Still be their parent, but not with micromanaged pressures we may have felt from our parents. To allow our children to step into their power, we must give them permission to do so. Young adults know that creating thousands of dollars of debt for college tuition doesn't work for everybody anymore, especially if they are unsure about what they want to do. Remember, just because our path or way did or did not work for us does not mean it may or may not work for them.

Sometimes with the allowance also comes failure. But just like when our children are first learning to walk, we cannot be there every step of the way to make sure they do not fall, and the same goes for their chosen path.

Failure is said to be one of the greatest teachers ever, and if you're reading this book, I am sure you too have failed. We, as parents, must welcome failure, just as we must be there to help them back up again.

I understand as a parent, we would do anything to keep a tear from running out of our kid's eyes, but this is part of our growth as much as theirs. There is no weakness in tears but merely a natural response of healing and honoring emotion.

Being a single father for almost the entirety of my daughter's life has been extremely difficult for me. The first couple of years after our divorce, I didn't communicate much at all with my ex. I learned to do my daughter's hair from YouTube and learned everything else from asking my mom or sisters.

As previously mentioned, my ex-wife is a wonderful mother. My daughter is definitely a mama's girl. As long as she knows I am always present, she is still safe and can always depend on me; that's all that truly matters. (Even though I do hope to sway her on the side of being a daddy's girl one day.)

Let me tell you where I failed. The hindrance of progression with her when she was younger. I allowed my depression, my pain, and my darkness to be projected upon her without even realizing it. I controlled my yelling, anger, and aggression, but my immense heaviness and sadness took a toll to the point where my daughter, a toddler, was worried about my well-being. How pitiful is that? I was so unaware of how I projected my energy that this young, innocent, beautiful soul became overly concerned of her depressed father. Even though I corrected myself, it still shouldn't have been an issue. If I knew then what I know now, it never would've happened.

This is why working on identification, setting intentions, taking responsibility, and being accountable for your actions to begin the healing process to obtain our true selves is the most important work we will ever embark on. Imagine how far the ripple can flow.

The article "Parental Depression" published by *Child Trends* (2018) stated,

"Parental depression negatively affects fathers' and mothers' caregiving, material support, and nurturance, and is associated with poor health and developmental outcomes for children of all ages, including prenatally. Children of depressed mothers are more likely than other children to have behavior problems, academic difficulties, and health problems (including psychiatric illness). According to another study, depressed fathers were less likely to engage their child in activities, and more likely to exhibit stress/aggravation in parenting."

This article provides a substantial amount of data and research that supports the effects parents can have on children if not taken care of immediately. Our energy immensely affects our children, and the effects of our projected energy can intensify at different ages of their lives.

My intention is not to scare you but to offer you understanding of how we are responsible for taking the proper steps to heal. This is a drastic understatement. We already know how much it has affected us day in and day out. Our pain can blind us to who we may be significantly hurting around us.

Family is the most important thing to me in my world, and I am sure it is in yours as well. "It's okay to become the hero of your story," Joe Rogan said, "and no longer the victim and subordinate to your past." Take time to look around to see how far your energy has spread, both positive and negative. Now do everything possible to remedy what needs to be corrected.

With this pain and darkness, it is easy to forget it is just not us feeling it. In some cases, it is spreading onto those we hold most dear.

I had to remember I could not be saved or have the work done for me by those who loved me. Do not become dependent upon your partner or your children to make you happy and find actual value within yourself. Just as you are not responsible for them in this manner, they are not responsible for you.

What a great opportunity you have to teach them from your experience as you carry on with your journey, so they will not have to suffer in the ways you unfortunately have.

Take the time each day and after each situation to evaluate the good and the bad. Notice where you can improve and where to have conversations for all in a safe, equal environment.

We must stop assuming everything will improve on its own as parents. Reflect every day with the intentions of betterment of self and solidarity of family.

We hear all the time that if we want to change the world, it starts within the doors of our own home. This ultimately falls on the shoulders of us parents.

If you are a parent who shares custody of your children, remove the ego and snarkiness that is only inhibiting your children's growth. Find a way to better communicate and co-parent with your ex. Create an opportunity for forgiveness and leave space for friendship once again. There is nothing more healing than allowing your children to see their parents in a healthy relationship.

You are no longer allowed to fall back on old ways of parenting or co-parenting. It's okay and necessary to create space for the difficult conversations we are all so used to avoiding.

There is nothing more humbling than parenting and sharing custody of a child. Work together in an upward and forward direction with your ex-partner. Become revolutionary in creating a new family unit and leave the old and toxic ways behind.

There is no greater reward than becoming the parent you are meant to be! Therefore, honor the process to do so and watch not only yourself shift but your entire family shift also.

VI

*"To run away from trouble is a form of cowardice and,
while it is true that the suicide braves death, he does it
not for some noble object but to escape some ill."*
Aristotle

My smile has always been one of my greatest attributes. People often complimented my smile but follow it up with, "Why don't you smile more?"

I had become a victim of my story, and my pain has become my foremost facial expression. I hid behind a scowl, even when I felt happy or apathetic. The face of anger and confusion was always present. With my larger-than-average presence and darker complexion, I warded off a lot of people. I had suppressed everything inside of me because I was so scared to be seen. Fear of being made fun of, fear of not being good enough, and fear of constant rejection plagued me.

Fear played right into my trauma. My fear of being judged for my race and past allowed people to judge me openly. It was all I thought about; therefore, it regularly manifested in my reality because that was precisely what I was projecting.

I rarely spoke to strangers. In groups, I was always quiet and reserved, which made me appear arrogant to many. Sadly, I just wanted people to see me, to get to know the real me, rather than intimidate them or create negative stories in my head after each interaction.

I had experienced so much pain in my life, I wasn't even sure how to process or make sense of it all. I just threw the next heartbreak, next failure, next disappointment in a bag and continued to lug it around everywhere I went.

I equate unhealed trauma and pain to a pregnant woman, and as a fitness professional, I feel comfortable using this analogy since I interact with pregnant women often. I don't mean to pinpoint any one person. This is just an observation of mine I've seen countless times.

Some women will get pregnant, not exercise at all during their pregnancy and gain a lot of weight on top of their baby weight. They will give birth, wait a couple years without regular exercise and get pregnant again, gaining more and more unwanted weight. This cycle continues for x number of babies, depending on the family. They will then come to me and ask to employ my expertise.

So what is the point I'm trying to make? All of us will or have experienced trauma or pain in our lives, but what so many of us do not do is heal from the experiences after they have passed. We continue to accumulate burden after burden and pack them down with each subsequent encounter. We carry these burdens to our next relationship and wonder why our relationship still doesn't work. We take the trauma to our next job and wonder why we aren't fulfilled, why we don't get along with our supervisors and coworkers. We wonder why close and personal friendships begin to deteriorate. Meanwhile, we place the blame on others.

When in reality, we're the ones out of alignment, and this spiral has now become a plague in our lives. We search endlessly for blame and to justify our actions. Even if we find it, we realize it still doesn't change our current condition. Which, in turn, makes us angrier. We then begin to wear it on our face, and the desire to show who we really are to the world is not even an option on the table anymore. Our pain has become our identity, and just like an overweight person, the excess weight severely limits everything we do.

All I wanted was to be seen. For people to see my huge heart rather than to be judged by my appearance. How could I do that when my anger overshadowed my eternal hope of being seen? I didn't do these things to myself! I didn't have a drug or addiction problem! I wasn't asked to be born to a mother that didn't want or care for me! I didn't ask to be placed in an environment that didn't accept me because of my race! I didn't ask for my dreams of playing football to be ripped out from under me because of a car accident that wasn't my fault! The world fucking owes me! Not the other way around!!

This was my mindset. I had become the ultimate definition of a victim.

So how did I change all that? How did I pivot my belief in my story? Ultimately, I didn't have a choice. The problem with becoming the victim is that you project negative energy everywhere, day in and day out. People can feel it, and even your closest friends and family start to avoid you. It's not because they don't love you or want the best for you, but you simply become an energy-sucking vampire, who takes away their progress, their happiness, and throws them out of alignment.

When we are in the epicenter of darkness, there is nothing but utter confusion, anger, sadness, and heartbreak. We cling to our trusted loved ones like leeches for any sense of guidance or relief from the heavy yoke we've been carrying.

I believe it is absolute desperation and survival skills that bring us to do this to those strong enough to be there, to take on some of that heaviness for us; there are no words which can express the gratitude we feel for you!

Although I deem myself an empath, and I feel I have carried a lot of weight for people around me, there are those who have carried an enormous burden for me. That is one of the purest forms of true love I have ever experienced.

Even so, there are times these people needed to create barriers and close themselves away from my energy, and that is an example of how you show up for yourself. Although you love those who are struggling, you still need to set boundaries and find the power in yourself to say no.

Because it also becomes painful and heavy for them, and if you are not an empath or one who experiences darkness and depression, it can be challenging to understand. In turn, it makes it hard for us to understand why and even feel abandoned when these barriers are created.

It was a hard lesson to learn, but now I understand. There is nothing wrong with communicating and asking before you unload your shit and energy on someone if they have space for you to unload. If not, space needs to be respected and allowed, and as so many of us know, it may be one of those terrible times we'll need to take it on by ourselves. This is a scary and lonely moment. But think how many times you have done it before, and you are still here fighting through it.

I implore anybody who is in a close relationship with someone who struggles with depression to educate themselves on how to best deal with and communicate in these situations. Realize you don't and can't always be the savior for these people, even though you may want to. You can, however, become knowledgeable on how to handle the situation in a way that is better for them and for yourself. Find power in loving yourself and still be able to show up for those you love with a completely different mindset of understanding.

There are times I reflect and wonder how the hell I have made it this far. How did I never succumb to the demons plaguing me every waking day of my life? Feeding me every reason and every excuse to end it! Why put up with this pain any longer? Why fight for a life most assuredly I wasn't meant to be living? Ego, perhaps?

We are always told ego is the enemy, and ego will impede us from our best selves and ward off that which is better for us, and I agree 99.9 percent. But for one instance, it was my ego that saved my life.

I wanted to be done with it. Every expectation had failed me, every ounce of hope had diminished, and the heaviness of mental anguish was now surging through my entire body. Panic attacks had become more rampant, my social skills had diminished completely, and there was nothing else to live for.

When you reach a point of such turmoil and pain, there is no conscious thought of those you would leave behind or the suffering your lack of existence would create for others. All I know is I wanted the pain to end.

A couple of years before what I'm about to tell you happened, I lost one of my closest friends to suicide. Until recently, I don't think I had given myself allowance to forgive myself for it.

For years, he would lean on me when he needed help understanding his dark and heavy days. I undertook that role with honor and gratitude. If anyone understood the deep pain he experienced, it was me.

We would get together often and continuously keep in contact, and just when I was at the point of beginning to worry about him, he met an angel of a woman. I couldn't be happier for him, and as I did, he carried a lot of his heaviness into that relationship. To my knowledge, she and their relationship had become his saving grace.

We would get together when time permitted, and he always seemed happier than ever. Before, he always seemed to be sick since I knew him, but a couple years into his marriage, all that changed. He was healthy, in better shape, and glowing.

Then one day, a mutual friend called me to let me know he had taken his life, and like all those who receive this dreadful call, I was in disbelief. How the hell did this happen? He was doing so well! He had a family. Why did he not reach out to me!? He knew I was there for him.

Like all that experience this, we do a great job of making it about ourselves and taking responsibility for something that was never our responsibility to bear.

He was one of the greatest friends and men I will ever know, but as you will soon see, I understand why he never threw out a lifeline to me.

Two summers after his passing, I returned from my yearly humanitarian trip to Africa, where I made quite a spectacle of myself by suffering from a mental breakdown.

I learned most humanitarian trips in third-world countries will show you all your shit in the most public way possible. After three consecutive years, I was no exception. My life had come to its tipping point, and I had reached my ultimate wits' end.

After I made a show for all to see, I called the airline and booked a ticket to leave eight days early, to no longer spin out of control in front of everybody and ruin their experience.

On the plane ride home, I planned it all. I planned where, how, and when. I was actually quite excited about it.

The day after I got home, and I had got my bearings back about me, I decided it was time. There is a spot that looks over the entire valley where I always would go to clear my thoughts and work through shit on my own. It had become a sacred place to me even though it was in a business section and not nearly secluded as I would've liked.

It was near the end of July, and dusk had just set in. I had driven and parked my car in the same spot I always do. I wrote a letter those most important to me and something a little bit more personal to my daughter, feeling her world would be so much better without me.

This time, I shed no tears or felt self-pity, just a motivation to end the 35 years of absolute misery I had experienced. I looked over the valley one last time and held the 9mm pistol to my right temple, and just as I did, a simple thought went through my head, "*Once you do this, you will forever regret it, and all hope will be gone.*" Call it my subconscious, call it a whisper from an angel, name it whatever you like, but immediately I put the gun down back under my seat. My ego immediately took over and said, "Fuck that!" The chip on my shoulder sounded! "I will not lose to myself today!"

Before I left the parking lot, I made myself one promise. If I put the gun down, I was never allowed to pick it up again. There would be no more back and forth, toiling with the idea of suicide again.

I drove home as if nothing out of the ordinary happened. A little confused because the pain and darkness were still present, I knew I could no longer be the victim; I had not only to fight but fight for self-healing.

The following day, I called my best friend, who had been one of my rocks. We met for lunch. He was more relieved than I was but also upset, and rightfully so.

After lunch, he pulled his car up to mine, and I gave him my gun. I still have not seen it to this day.

Humans are hardwired to place judgments on things we don't understand. For those lucky enough to never have battled depression or suicidal thoughts, know we who do suffer would ultimately do anything to end the pain and anguish we suffer from to the point of taking our own lives to do so.

It was so imperative for me to look at all the factors that led me to the point of suicide.

Dr. Galynker explained in an article published by *The New York Times*, "What people experience before attempting suicide is a combination of panic, agitation, and franticness. A desire to escape from unbearable pain and feeling trapped." (2015)

This statement couldn't be more profound. My pain wasn't something that came and went like the weather but was a constant weight inside of me that I couldn't shake, and I had absolutely no idea there were tools out there to improve myself. If the painful emotions are not directed out, a tipping point is inevitable.

I had not known or understood the power of breathing and the fantastic effect it has during panic attacks. It allows me to center myself and think within myself rather than entering into the chaos outside my head. Six simple, intentional, deep breaths gave me the power and peace during the most turbulent of storms. You have the means to ease any storm that enters your space if you are willing to learn how to use the tools to get you to a state of calm.

If you are willing to set a new positive intention every day, you will be able to change the current direction of any aspect of your life, but it must be followed with consistent practice, and you must transform the thought into action. Your action must be accompanied by accountability.

Check yourself when the negativity enters, pull yourself out of your own negative patterns, rather than just allowing them to take over.

Reach out to a close friend or coach who can help keep you accountable and honest. Next, you need to move out of victim mode. Quit playing the toxic blame game. Remember the moment you take responsibility for your current situation will give you the grit and power to begin the work. If you are continually pointing fingers to blame others for your problems, you will stay immobile and without purpose. Honestly, not many people want to hear over and over why you are losing.

Chris Rock said, "I'd always end up breaking down on the highway. When I stood there trying to flag someone down, nobody stopped. But when I pushed my own car, other drivers would get out and push with me. If you want help, help yourself—people like to see that."

Those closest around you cannot do the work for you! No matter how much they love you and would like to stand in for you. It can't be done. Just like nobody can go to the gym for you to shed off the extra pounds. Pick up your tools and begin to work, then you will be amazed at the support system that begins to grow around you.

Mental illness definitely gave me a type of entitlement during my victimization. I believed that not only did the world owe me by making things right but my friends and family also did. When I finally realized nobody was coming to save me, I had to set my ego aside and take all the responsibility for my shit. It was humbling, yet again, it was part of the process.

I had to give myself permission. Permission to heal and do the work. Permission to forgive myself for this position I was in. Permission to forgive my inner child, and permission to never ever quit!

I am not going to tell you the same old cliché of *what doesn't kill you makes you stronger*. I don't honestly believe that rhetoric, but what I do believe is all the horrible storms you have weathered give you the ripe opportunity to become wiser. There is a lesson and a balance in all things, good and bad. It just depends entirely on where you would like to focus your lens and direct your energy.

During the chaos of our downward spiral, we tend to self-sabotage and sometimes make these situations much worse than they need to be. We make irrational decisions, so we may appear to be a bigger victim than we already are. In a sense, we become drama queens. Paranoia and fear creep in to help our stories become even more grandiose than actual reality. Rational thought goes to shit, and there we are, buckled in for another ride to Fuck Town.

These patterns will continue until we are the ones willing to shift away from them and our old beliefs are released.

You may find conflict inheriting a new belief system. Second-guessing yourself when you have found comfort in old wounds and darkness. Do not let this turn you away from continuing to learn and incorporate sound, practical healing methods.

So many of us stay in a mess of sadness because we feel there is no other way to live life and handle whichever situations this world has brought upon us. We have programmed ourselves to think, believe, and feel this is the only way, and in fact, that is simply the program you are running.

There is another way. There are many other different modes of thinking, believing, and feeling. One only needs to be willing to learn and upload them to the conscious mind.

You are the victim as long as you continue to choose to be the victim. You will lose only as long as you consciously decide to lose. Until you decide to change that frame of mind into victory and the onset of winning, nothing can be changed.

Stop waiting for the perfect day, time, or event to begin. The timing will never be perfect, and chances are, when you do start, you might be thrown another curveball.

I had to create the mindset that once I set my gun down, I could never pick it back up again. Nor could I again wallow in the fantasies of suicide. Would I still feel the urge of darkness beckoning me back to my habitual loathsome patterns? Absolutely! But I fought with the same sort of tenacity and charge as I did when I was running a football or rugby ball. I'd get my ass knocked down and get back up. There was no other choice, and there is no other choice for you when you choose to create a new vision for yourself.

For those in the fight of your lives, I ask that you keep fighting. I ask you to keep seeking what helps you. Understand there is a path for you to find your way out of the dark.

I am sorry you feel so alone, and the weight upon you has become so unbearable. Keep fighting! And you will soon find your way!

Pay attention to each day and every action you are committing. Are your habits forthcoming with each goal and destination you've set for yourself? Are you able to catch yourself loathing in your circumstances? If so, can you shift away?

Begin to take hold of your habits. Recognize the ones pulling you down and away from your path. Replace them with more positive ones.

Find power in speaking mantras of all the great things you want and where you would like to be into existence. Be specific with each one. Counter each negative thought with a positively charged affirmation.

I've been asked before how I knew if I was healing. How did I know if the work I was undertaking is genuinely helping? What I have discovered for myself is when you can share your story and experiences of your past traumas, you do not become emotional, resentful, numb, or victimized. Instead, you have a sense of empowerment. A feeling of, "YES, I experienced that shit, and look how fucking amazing I am on the other side!"

You have removed yourself from being a slave to what once was and are all-powerful to what now is because you have completely shifted into alignment with your higher and authentic self.

As you continue to heal, you will begin to look back and see how certain instances that once bothered you no longer do. You will see triggers have lessened their effect on you.

For me, much of my pain and traumas are still very recent, while some are very old. Scars are just beginning to heal, and others mended long ago, but my perception of them is far different than what I saw in the past. I am now humbly proud of what I have been through. I was able to lean into myself like never before, and I was able to do this for myself, by myself.

For some, it takes a mighty occurrence to push us to our knees. For others, it's a plethora of events that help us understand what we must do.

However, you are being called to heal and take your power back. Do it now and wait no longer!

Become mindful of what can be learned and implemented for you and those around you. Take the pain and now push it into wisdom. Take the anger and charge it into forward energy and take the attitude of "why me'" and throw it out the window. Because it has not and will never serve you.

To find the power, you must speak it into existence, and each spoken word must be spoken with grand ferocity. Allow your entire body to feel everything you would like to manifest into your reality. There is no more room for half-hearted emotion or pessimistic afterthought.

You have been summoned to the battle of your life. Answer the call!

VII

"We all have this misunderstanding about heartbreak, which is we think we should avoid it. But what I think is heartache is a clue towards the work we're supposed to be doing in the world. What breaks each person's heart is different - be racial injustice, war, or animals. And when you figure out what it is that breaks yours, go toward it."
Glennon Doyle Melton

It had been three years since my divorce when I finally hit my stride. My ex and I were still trying to figure things out when it came to being single again and co-parenting, but I felt we were on par with what's to be expected.

I began to heal in my heart, and slowly, I began to feel as though I could trust again.

I had been seeing one girl in particular. We had started off as friends, and then over a couple years, she became one of my most entrusted persons in my life, even though I couldn't possibly see a future with her or with any girl at that time.

I shunned every opportunity that gave rise to relationship talks and did my best to keep her at arm's length. Because of the heartbreak and disappointment I felt from my marriage, I was still very cautious about moving forward with anybody in the future.

We had been dating off and on, all while openly dating other people. We would talk about who we dated and how it was going. We asked each other for advice and how we would handle each situation.

Although we spent most of our time together, I made sure we came without a label. No commitment and no obligation.

Until one day, the dreaded "well" came.

We were vacationing in Mexico with some friends. During our last night at dinner, she suddenly asked, "Well, what's going on with us?" It was a question I knew that was coming, but I also was doing everything in my power to avoid it. I first took it as a joke, hoping a smug reply would knock this conversation away. It didn't. Then her tears came. She exclaimed she knew she wanted to be with me, and she had enough time waiting around. I either needed to commit to this relationship or else after this trip, it was a wrap. I continued to laugh it off, not because I wanted to hurt her, but because I had no idea how to react in this situation. I knew I sincerely cared for her, but in all of my relationships before her, I always ended up hurting my partner. Not out of betrayal or deceit but because I protected my heart by locking it up.

Even if I wanted to open up and commit, I had no idea how. I ended up telling her I cared for her, but right then, I still wasn't ready, which I wasn't.

The following day I returned home while she stayed behind for work. On the plane ride home, I couldn't help but wonder if I made a grave mistake. She was beautiful, super funny, and successful. We liked the same things, so what exactly was holding me back? Here's where it gets interesting.

When she returned from her trip, I raced over to her house to let her know how horrible of a mistake I made, and I wanted to take her up on her offer. I wanted to try things out and see if we could make it work.

What caught me off guard is she had already checked out. She was over it, but could I blame her? She bore her heart to me, and I laughed at her.

After a long conversation, the roles were completely reversed. She was no longer trying to talk me into the relationship; I was trying to talk her into one.

I realize now that I wasn't trying to win her back out of love but out of fear. I was afraid I was going to lose our friendship, which I greatly cherished. I was fearful that any potential of a meaningful relationship was long lost.

After a bit of coaxing, I finally swayed her back to the idea of being together, but first, she was going to Las Vegas on an all-girls' trip. Fucking Vegas!

She had gone to Las Vegas before, and it never bothered me. I guess before I never had any skin in the game like I did then. We had kept in contact while she was away, but upon her return, something felt different; something felt off. I asked her if anything happened, and she assured me nothing did. She was just so happy that she finally had me as a boyfriend, according to her.

For some reason, I couldn't believe her. Something deep inside me was calling her bluff, and the night she returned, I told her I couldn't be in the relationship. I didn't believe that nothing happened, and my gut was telling me to close the door and move on.

A couple of days later, I left for Africa with a humanitarian group. We decided to meet when I returned to discuss what was to come next for us. My time in Africa flew by, and I found myself again questioning my decision and thinking about this girl often.

When I arrived home, she texted me and said she needed to talk. I wasn't worried but curious about what she had to say. I knew she hadn't moved on, and I thought she would tell me more about her Las Vegas trip. I jumped on the phone with her, and she told me that she had met someone and that if it were okay with me, she'd like to see where things went with him.

Honestly, I wasn't mad or even upset about it. I was definitely caught off guard.

Looking back, I realized it did wound my ego a bit, but emotionally, I thought I was genuinely okay. Until I saw them together.

That's when it struck me and struck me hard. I guess it never affected me until it entered my three-dimensional reality. I was on my way to work at the gym when I saw her and her new dude drive right by me. It was then I realized she was gone, and I had fucked up.

Or so I thought.

I don't necessarily remember what took me there, but before I knew it, I was texting and calling her, doing everything I could to get her back. I had lost all my power, and I had become entirely vulnerable. Something I promised myself I would never do again.

I soon found out this new guy was already living with her or at least staying with her. That broke me for two reasons.

One, because I did not realize how much of myself I had given to her.

I was in absolute gut-wrenching pain, and at times I couldn't even breathe.

Two, because she had moved on so fast. Everything I thought we had invested, and I thought we had planted some form of foundation, was entirely a lie! (See the pattern of thinking here yet?)

A few days later, I persuaded her to meet me late one night in a 24 Hour Fitness parking lot. That was it. I was going to beg her back. Forget pride, forget dignity. I groveled before her, crying for the first time since my marriage. It was funny because I had dropped this facade of over-confidence. I had broken every promise I made to myself. Specifically, that I would never become vulnerable before a woman again. I had written a story in my head that every woman, including my birth mother, had betrayed me in one way or another. Here I was, in full desperation mode, about to feel this too familiar feeling of abandonment once again.

I know she was as surprised as I was. Surprised to see a man who was once incapable of any outside emotion fall in defeat of a broken heart, and I did!

She shared tears as well, crying she didn't know what she was doing, and she never would've done it if only I told her how I really felt in Mexico. Looking back, I realize that was my chance, and this situation was really my fault.

After a few days of calls and a lot of texting, she said the guy staying with her was leaving, and it obviously wasn't working out.

She wanted to try and work things out if only my sorry ass could forgive her. (I added the sorry ass.) You'll soon find out why.

I immediately jumped at the opportunity to take her up on her offer. All I wanted was not to feel whatever fucked up feelings permeated through me.

It was a constant feeling deep inside the pit of my stomach, like you feel when you're standing right on the edge of a tall cliff or building, and all I wanted to do was get rid of it.

We started hanging out like old times. This time things had changed significantly. She had immediately become secretive. Texting in the other room and putting the phone face down whenever we were together. What was the hell going on? I knew these signs. I knew exactly what was going on, but I justified it. I justified all of it. It didn't matter; I just wanted her back.

A couple days later, I was working out with a good friend who was playing with the Miami Dolphins at the time. Between sets, he asked if I still saw what's-her-name. Automatically I could feel a bombshell coming, so I answered vaguely. He said, "Last time I was in town, I saw her at the club. She was at my table all night and then came home to my hotel room. We had a good night." He immediately saw the expression on my face change.

I couldn't hide it.

He continued on, "Shit, I fucked up, didn't I? Man, I didn't know. Man, I'm sorry."

I wasn't mad at him; I'll never be mad at him. Even if he did know. I replied, "No, man, you did me a favor." Everything about that entire relationship was like driving my car the wrong way on the freeway. I was on a collision course, making an irrational decision because I refused to listen to my heart and gut instinct, simply because I put my ego and fear first before any rational thinking.

What was funny about that situation was that I knew precisely the night it happened. I remembered a few events were going on throughout the Valley the night she hooked up with my friend, and I was hoping to get together with her, but she told me she was sick and going to bed. I never questioned her. I had no reason to think otherwise.

After finding out about her indiscretion, I called her right as I left the gym; I shouted a few choice words and left that story forever in my past.

But remember earlier how I shared that something was more than off when she went to Vegas? It just so happens that the very guy who was staying with her turned out to be the man she eventually married.

Now I can look back with real joy and happiness that she found her match.

Most of us have had a great heartbreak story. Usually, heartbreak happens because we choose to justify recurring patterns. We wish only to see what we want to know because we could never believe the person we love and uphold would do such a horrible thing to us. No matter what our friends and family tell us and warn us, we believe we can change them. We assume they will love us enough to make us work and never break us in the process. And we've seen this story over and over in our lives. In our personal lives and within our social circles.

Some of us choose to drive the wrong way on the freeway, thinking by some miracle, all of the traffic will redirect itself and conform to our outrageous direction. Then we drive head-on into a semi-truck.

Like most athletes, I have experienced my fair share of devastating injuries. From ACL tears, broken ribs, to torn AC joints in both shoulders. All of them have paled in comparison to heartbreak and betrayal. Not to mention the cataclysmic feeling of being abandoned once again!

As time and healing went on, it was interesting to look back at this relationship and identify the parts where I went wrong. I learned to see how I was responsible for the outcomes once the fog of pain and confusion cleared. It was here I was able to reflect upon where I was guilty of these heart-wrenching consequences.

Being single in this day and age differs significantly from the generations before us. We live in a time where commitment and accountability have become more of a guideline than an honorable pact to uphold. Social media has surged so dramatically it has trained our mind there is always better, and we can do better.

Many choose not to share if they're in an exclusive relationship for two reasons.

First, because they don't want the rest of the world following their private business, which I can understand.

Second, just in case there is that one chance something better comes along, or their long-awaited crush becomes single, they don't want to appear in a committed relationship.

So when I look back and openly see my guilt, I see I never fully committed to her.

Even though I wasn't doing it to see what was better out there, I was doing it to protect myself so I could heal correctly and not hurt her as I had previously done to other girls.

Even though she was doing her own thing behind my back when I was thinking we were on a completely different page, she was within her own right to do what she did. All the while, she continually brought up the conversation of "what were we?"

I realize in her eyes, I was more of a conquest rather than a commitment, and that's okay. She needed that validation, just as many of us do in the dating life.

So I ask you now, Are you always looking to be validated by a partner? To conquer the next challenge? To fulfill your ego, thinking it'll make you feel better? Prettier? More desirable?

I am speaking to both men and women here. Please, don't get me wrong. The single life can be fun. Especially when we take the right time and path to heal and become more aware of what it is precisely we're looking for.

But not at the expense of causing the same traumas that were committed against us. I'm guilty of it, as so many of us are, but I was able to catch myself and realize the damage I was causing. Then I took a timeout from dating altogether. I gave myself time to realize what it was that kept me locking my heart up so tight.

Where were my blind spots I could improve upon to make me a more suitable, healthy partner?

Unfortunately, right here is where it gets tricky.

How many of us are or know somebody who can't be alone? They go from one relationship to the next within weeks, and the cycle never stops.

Instead of taking the great opportunity to gather themselves, reflect, learn, and heal, they emotionally shit on the next person in their dating pool.

What's the common factor after each relationship comes to a blistering end? Yes, that's right! They believe they are the victims, and it is always the other person's fault.

One of the greatest blessings we can have is taking and upholding the opportunity to stand alone. To go deep within ourselves. To feel into whatever pain it is that is drowning us from a clear vision of what we want and how we need to be loved.

To get to know who we truly are. To seek, to find, and to align.

So many of us fail when presented with this opportunity. Why? Perhaps it's past trauma, or the thought of being alone scares the shit out of us. So we choose to be stuck in the same loop over and over, living the same story of insanity. This causes more trauma and pain to us and those whom we want to date and attempt to love.

The moment we choose to take the time to heal is the moment where our power is revealed.

We only have one chance at this life; isn't it time that we get to know ourselves for the first time to see how great we truly are? To maximize every ounce of waking potential we have?

Stop living the current program you are running and dive deep into yourself.

This part of my life continues to be my greatest battle for me to overcome.

I have allowed the effects of being an abandoned baby have too much impact on my life. I can reflect back and see how much I clung to women, needing to fill that empty space I didn't even know existed. I took this trauma into my marriage unknowingly and also brought it into the relationship I have now.

Because of this mindset, we almost didn't make it this far several times.

My inherent fear of being abandoned was always present, and that trigger still goes off. After my divorce, I had become more confident in myself than I ever had in my entire life. Looking back now, I see this confidence was also a facade because my heart and emotions were completely turned off. I had become unaffected by any pain because I was numb, which most therapists would say is worse than feeling pain.

For me, I was careless in how I made my decisions and very insensitive to the feelings of others.

Heartbreak, no matter who it happens to, takes a long time to recover from. We replay the situations over and over in our mind and ask ourselves what we did to deserve this.

We feel stupid, played, and confused. Then we begin to question ourselves. The horrible feeling of rejection. Our self-confidence and esteem are completely diminished to nothing.

We can't eat, we can't sleep, and we obsess about what the other person is doing and who they are doing it with.

We are left wishing there was a special antidote that we could take to end the physical, emotional, and mental anguish that comes with heartbreak, but there isn't any.

I am not going to tell you time heals everything because that's not entirely true. What rings true is what you decide to do with your time, and no, I don't recommend going on a tirade by sleeping with any and everybody. But after you're done sulking and crying every minute of the day, you will start to feel stronger little by little.

I want you to evaluate yourself in terms of your relationship the same way your boss would at your year-end review. Ask yourself these questions:

Would you date you, knowing the shit you are carrying? If so, are you working each day consciously with the purpose to identify and heal from your shit?

Has my heartbreak come from dating the same type of person over and over? If so, am I willing to pivot in a new direction?

Have I taken the time to really and truly love and know myself?

Do I know my worth? Like, really fucking KNOW MY WORTH?

Will I need constant validation from my partner to feel loved?

After assessing these questions honestly and truthfully, you'll know whether or not to proceed.

What I realize is the only people who seem to be immune to heartbreak are those who refuse to give their heart away, and that's a sad case all on its own.

We are going to fall; we are going to feel broken and shattered like we never thought we were capable of feeling. Now I realize all the struggles were worth going through to find the partner I have today. To experience the love, loyalty, understanding, and power of a partner who truly sees me, and I see her.

Take the time to learn from the mistakes you have made in relationships. Be honest with yourself about whichever expectations you have.

Know what you are deserving of, but first, make sure you are worthy of yourself. Find power in loving who you are and who you have become.

Be willing to become aware of your shit and your triggers, but also know you do not need to be entirely perfect and healed before you go off to find your partner. Chances are this person will help catapult you in the very direction you need and keep you motivated to do the work.

This is why who you select as a partner and alignment with yourself are so important. Because you will accept nothing less than someone on this very same path with you.

The absolute fears of abandonment still haunt me to this day, as well as the fear of being betrayed and having the ugly ghost of heartbreak visit me once again. The difference between then and now is that I can identify my triggers. I can speak about them out loud and work through them rather than pitfall into a never-ending chasm, and that is the work. This is the work!

We will never be completely free of all of our traumas and fears, but we can gain the ability to identify them and see them from a different perspective. Understanding that our fears are stories we have created in our head gives us control of deciding how much power we choose to give them. The more we understand our fear, the more we can control it. Or, we can yield power over to fear to the damning point of actualization, regardless of whether the stories are true or not. We can also have the ability to see what is occurring in our minds and cast fear out.

Remember, light was created out of darkness, and because of these immense times of peril, one can be the sole creator of whom they'd like to become.

Do not be afraid of getting to know yourself and consider even dating yourself.

There will come a time when your exes' choices can no longer dictate who you are and where you are going.

Become sufficient and resilient in how you proceed away from heartbreak. The point isn't only moving away from your pain but not passing on that same exact pain to others. By doing so, you create the grounds for those worthy of your attention, who will value you, as you now value yourself.

There is no fear in self-love but utter confusion in a lost identity created by how we feel others view us.

VIII

"The truth is: Belonging starts with self-acceptance. Your level of belonging, in fact, can never be greater than your level of self-acceptance, because believing that you're enough is what gives you the courage to be authentic, vulnerable and imperfect."
Brene Brown

I never truly understood the severity of my depression until I went to college. I had so many expectations and hoped to finally become part of a group where I would be accepted. I was so exhausted from doing everything I could to fit in during my junior high and high school years, I was finally ready to be around my kind of people, and by my kind, I mean people of color.

Though I was genuinely grateful for my new friends, I know they could never understand what it was like for me to grow up in the same environment as I did.

I remember one of the first weeks of football practice, the team was running passing routes. I went in and lit it on fire. I ran routes on senior defensive backs that were never expected from a true freshman. Shoot, I was surprising myself. It was right then and there when I realized I perform better under pressure and feel I have something to prove because that is how I had been living my entire life.

Before that first practice session, I was greatly intimidated and expected to be humbled by superior players, but that wasn't the case at all. I had left my mark that day, and now for the first time in my life, I was ready to be accepted by my own.

Unfortunately, that wasn't what played out. My short, brief career in college football, scorched with injury after injury due to a previous car wreck, didn't leave me with a bunch of brothers like I hoped.

Because I'm multiracial, many people do not know what to make of me at first glance. Was I Polynesian? Filipino? Black and White? For the majority of my life, I hated that people didn't know I was half black. I had suffered so much racism growing up. I felt that I finally could "wear my color" with pride.

I didn't come from the ghetto or inner city like the majority of my teammates. I didn't identify with black culture, only that of what I had seen on TV or in the movies. I shined on the field when I was healthy, which was a rarity, and I was quickly labeled "the square" or "whitewashed" among my peers. It appeared my last hope of fitting in and being accepted was gone.

While at college, most of my friends from high school had left on a two-year church mission. It was then, in my freshman year, I realized I was all alone once again. Being out of touch with old friends and not being easily accepted by new friends was a difficult combination to comprehend. I attached myself to the belief that I would become part of a new fraternity of men who identified and understood what it was to be a man of color, and they would accept me like my long-lost family.

The friends I hung out with on the team happened to be white, and as it were, I identified with them more because of my cultural upbringing. So again, because of the disappointment, feeling of rejection, and not feeling like I belonged reinforced the emotional and mental pain I felt in my past.

During this time in my life, like so many of us at this age, I had no idea how to process my feelings. I wasn't even aware there were outlets and other ways to work through this pain. All I know is it became way too much to bear.

So, I started cutting myself. I don't know how I started, but all I know is that it temporarily took away the pain.

I would always cut my left wrist or shoulder and cut deep enough to make myself bleed. Sometimes deeper than other times. I had a couple teammates notice because I didn't cover the cuts. I would simply laugh it off and say that it was from being tackled on the turf.

I cut myself throughout my short career. This was the only time I did so. All I remember is the last time I cut myself, it hurt so much that I didn't do it again.

I realize now, I was doing this to feel once again. After 18 years of rejection and unidentified feelings of abandonment and confusion, I was numb to all emotions.

I would like to quote an article published in *Psychology Today* called "Self Injury: 4 Reasons Why They Cut and What to Do."

Reason #1: Physical pain takes away emotional pain. The physical pain of cutting not only diffuses negative emotion but it also creates a sense of calm and relief.

Reason #2: People who cut are their own harshest critics.

People who cut reported feeling dissatisfied with themselves much more often than non-cutters.

Reason #3: Cutting can be a way to stop feeling numb. In particular, individuals with a trauma history may self-harm to take control of their own pain and feel something other than numbness.

Reason #4: It's an alternative outlet for emotional pain.

They turn to cutting as an "acceptable" way to feel pain—if they're not allowed to feel it emotionally, they'll let it out physically.

The article continues with, "In short, think of cutting and self-harm as any other unhealthy coping mechanism like getting drunk, binge eating, or getting high; it's a way to feel something other than what you're feeling, or it can be a way to punish yourself for not measuring up." It took 15 years to realize the depth of my depression. However, my depression had plummeted much lower just a couple years ago.

So why didn't I reinitiate cutting as I did so long ago? First, because the thought of it disgusted me. Even though I may not have understood it thoroughly then, I have gained a much higher love and gratitude for the human body and its capabilities.

Second, because I had already made myself a promise after setting my gun down—not only could I never pick it up again, I couldn't do any more bodily harm whatsoever.

And third, because I realized I was on the radar of my close friends and family, they all noticed my struggle and were fearful for me. I didn't really care to set off another alarm louder than the ones already sounding off.

College flew by quickly. Due to the onset of injuries from my car accident, I decided to put my athletic career on hold. After talking to the coach and beginning my junior-year football season with another hamstring tear, we decided that I should take a two-year break and fulfill my obligations as a Christian by serving a two-year mission for the Church of Jesus Christ of Latter-Day Saints (also known as the Mormon church). The plan was that I would get two good years away from football to heal. Then I would come back to my scholarship, all rested up, and finish my career. Or so I thought.

For me, growing up Mormon and black in the state of Utah in the early 1980s was extremely difficult. In the late 1970s, the church allowed blacks to receive the same "blessings and callings" as the rest of the world's ethnicities and races. When this new law was passed, I was told it was celebrated by the majority of church members throughout the land, but it was also known hundreds showed up in downtown Salt Lake City to protest at church headquarters. So it was fair to say some did not like the thought of blacks equally being recognized in the church, and this way of thinking for many exists today.

I set out on my two-year obligation to fulfill my church responsibilities as a man. If I fulfilled this obligation honorably, the church "promised" that I would come back to an abundance of blessings, and so I did. I worked my ass off for the entirety of my two-year obligation.

About three months before I was due to return home, I received the news my coach was leaving for another school, and the promise of coming back to my scholarship was in jeopardy.

My dad quickly got on the phone to make sure my scholarship would be honored when I returned. The new coach was the old defensive coordinator whom I thought I had a good relationship with. Upon my arrival, he promised my dad I would be eligible for my scholarship, and my fear quickly dissipated.

The day after I arrived home, I met with the coach. "I'm sorry, Rob, but I can't give you your scholarship. I have a new coaching staff, and unfortunately, they don't know who you are. If you want to play here, you must prove your worth once again as a walk-on."

I can't say I was too surprised. Two years is a long time to be away from college football, especially right in the middle of a career. I guess I just hoped the coach would've been a little more candid with my dad on the phone.

I decided to walk on and do my best to remind them of the player I was. But that opportunity wasn't ever given. I was quickly put on the scout team and switched positions from running back to a receiver—a position I had never played in my life, but to be honest, I realized I wasn't the player I once was. During my two-year hiatus, I barely trained or maintained my athletic ability.

After camp was over and realizing I had a starting spot on the scout team and no scholarship, I reluctantly decided to part ways with the team.

Looking back on the situation, do I wish I stuck it out with the team and proved my worth once again? Sometimes.

Was my decision made directly by my ego? Absolutely! How could they not remember me? Does a promise not mean anything anymore? Don't we still honor our commitments as men? Very rarely.

High school sports, college, pros, it's all a business. After many years of processing, it's no longer my coach I am mad at or place blame. He is only given an allotted amount of scholarships each year, and me coming back was definitely a wild card.

The summer before starting my career in college football, I was driving a close friend home. As we pulled up to the intersection in a suburban neighborhood, I began to proceed through a green light to turn left, and the last thing I saw was flashing lights.

A cop car had run a red light and T-boned us on the left side at nearly 80 miles per hour as he was responding to a home invasion call.

Both my friend and I climbed out of the totaled Nissan Altima, and then I went immediately into shock.

As I lay there on the street, I remember the officer walking over and telling me sternly, "Get up, you're fine!" So I crawled over to the sidewalk, where I waited for the ambulance.

I suffered a severe concussion and two herniated discs from the side impact, and my friend suffered severe whiplash and a concussion.

We are lucky to be alive and still walking today!

Unfortunately, the injury I sustained plagued me through my short tenure on the team. Being somewhat ignorant of the human body and how it heals, becoming sidelined was my new normal.

I was angry at the police officer and accident for so long. I trained so hard each off-season with high hopes and expectations that always turned into disappointments.

Having to come home to another kick-in-the-nuts quickly added to my narrative that the world is against me.

Years later, I decided to leave organized religion altogether. I never felt right or equal within the walls of the church. I always felt like an outsider.

While I practiced my faith, I was faithful. All I wanted to do is what I was taught was right. That was the environment in which I was thrown into and acclimated to. But, like all environments, it came with good and bad qualities.

Over time, I had constructed a belief system that wasn't my own. It wasn't at all conducive to who I was as a man of color, and it wasn't designed to serve me in my highest good.

I did not walk away with one bit of resentment or ill will towards the church. I am grateful for the moral compass it instilled in me, the family values it taught me, and the two years I served honorably.

I was taught so many lessons that significantly formed me into the man I am today.

I have seen many walk away and leave the church with such anger and malice in their heart because they feel they have been deceived.

They feel beguiled by what they once coveted with faith and devotion is now filled with hate.

Is this a beneficial trade? Is your newfound liberation genuinely liberating? Or perhaps have you found a new pair of shackles to replace the old? This can happen with any new belief system.

If you are plagued by anger or rage because you have chosen a new way of believing, a new god, or a new religion, but you hold contempt in your heart for what you once believed in, how can you possibly move forward in faith, power, or devotion when you are anchored with dark energy from your past?

Instead, look back with gratitude and appreciation for the great things that were learned and incorporated into your life and your family. If you focus solely on the dirt, then that is what your heart will become, entrenched with the very negative emotions you are trying to move away from.

If I can share anything from this lesson, it is to believe in what makes you happy, whether it's religion, spirituality, or yourself—if it makes you happy, believe in it!

Daily, I see people plagued with guilt and fear because of what they choose to believe in. Is that really living? Is that fulfilling our real purpose?

My truth is not your truth, and it doesn't have to be. Find your truth, magnify it, and live out your purpose.

As for me, like a lot of us, it wasn't until adulthood when I discovered my truth. I realized the programs running within me and around me weren't working. I was trying to force myself into a space where I didn't fit, which I don't blame anyone for.

I had to throw all my puzzle pieces back on the table, spread them around, and pick them up to see exactly how they fit together to create a life and a power which was for me. No more copying and pasting to blend in anymore, when I never really had anyways.

After college, it was apparent I didn't fit in anywhere. Not with whom I hoped, not with teammates, and most definitely not with my religious community.

It was then where my loneliness rolled in like a rogue wave. As I mentioned earlier, I did everything I could to fit in growing up, and it was then I realized there was no more faking it to make it.

Even though I longed to relate with brothers of color in ways I had been starving for, I knew, for now, that wouldn't be my tribe.

Years later, I came to the point and mindset where I no longer allowed my environment to dictate nor validate who I was as a man. Because of this, I fell into solitude. I took on the challenge to find myself for the first time in my life. Although at the time, it felt more mandated than chosen.

In hindsight, I realize if I were accepted among my fellow teammates in the manner that I was seeking, I know for certain I would've allowed them, or any group at that time, to define me as a man. Which is not entirely a bad thing, but I was vulnerable and so desperate to belong, my identity would be lost to them, and I would have no room for my true self to be realized.

Years after I left the football team, I still told everyone I met that I played football for the local university. Football was always a big part of my identity, and like so many fallen athletes, I had no idea how else to identify myself.

Throughout my professional career, I have worked with highly decorated retired military men, and upon their return also came a lost sense of identity.

They were used to walking in a room where everybody immediately fell silent, stood up, and saluted. That was the weight and respect they carried, but when they returned home, nobody was aware of what great sacrifices and courageous acts they committed. They were civilians again, with great stories to share for those who would lend an ear. Although my career was spotty and quickly over, in a small sense, I did understand the loss of identity because all I had ever known, and ever been, was a football player.

How many of us have allowed this to happen in our own lives? We have allowed our career to become our identity and define who we are as a man or woman. That's all we discuss on the first date, right? What do you do? Then we spout off whatever our current endeavor is and make it sound 10 times more glamorous than it really is.

Here is exactly where the work comes in. Your career is not who you are. Motherhood, fatherhood, your hobbies, your unique skills, your amazing world-record feats are still not who you are. Many of us have latched on to whatever is our most proud accomplishment and use that to describe the *what*. Perhaps because we never thought to dig a little deeper than the tangible outer layer of our existence. Or maybe we've never wanted to, for fear of what we may or may not find.

Remember, this world is scattered with too many distractions to prevent us from the foremost extraordinary accomplishment, which is finding ourselves.

Have you ever met somebody who spouts off their entire resumé and list of accomplishments without even being asked about it? At first, it comes off as very pompous and arrogant, right? What I have learned, as I have taken a step back, is that these people aren't only saying these things for me to hear and seem amazed by. They are verbally validating themselves as well. They have predicated their entire life's journey on the *what* rather than the *who*. Even if their doings are quite remarkable, it still doesn't show me who they are as a person, other than perhaps being a little arrogant.

It doesn't matter which program you are running. Religion, sports, tribe, career, politics. If you are not living for you and your conscious betterment, you are doing it wrong.

If you have the mindset and attachment of needing something other than yourself to validate or even quantitate your value as a person, then you must come to the harsh realization that self-trust and self-love have not been appropriated yet.

Now let me expound on this for those who reach for offense before they reach for understanding.

Obviously, being passionate about your hobbies, friends, family, or personal beliefs is enriching and even necessary for so many of us to have in our lives. If those things are truly making you happy and a better person, please continue engaging in them with full force. In order for your true identity and your true power of self to be realized, you must identify it from the inside.

If you continue to allow external factors to dictate your identity as a person, you cannot hold any stance with power. You will continue to depend on an external source for validation and how you deem yourself to the world.

Most people can see through that, even if it is not brought to your attention. It comes off vain and egotistical to those who honestly would like to know you and your story. Do not take those opportunities lightly.

If you want to be seen, then be willing to show yourself, but remove yourself from hiding behind your significant accomplishments, religious verses, and political jargon. There is a time and a place for all of those things. No longer be defined by *what*, so you can feel the power of you.

I am not a football player or a rugby player; I played those things. And I loved that I had the opportunity to do so, but I would hate if anyone ever introduced me as one because I am more than an accomplished athlete. If I was to be introduced to some of my more exceptional accomplishments, those labels are still not who I am. My tribe, my religion, my anything external is not who I am.

Come to love and accept yourself first, then your presence alone will dictate the rest—unsaid! The *what* around you will further compliment the person within you.

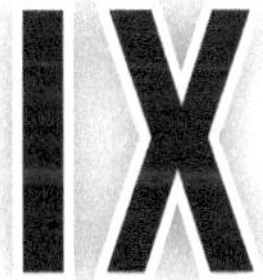

"Without great solitude, no serious work is possible."
Pablo Picasso

Spiritual awareness via solitude is an ancient tradition practiced throughout the world by different tribes and cultures for thousands of years. In many parts, one cannot become a man or woman until one has accomplished the ceremonial calling.

Imagine for a moment having no choice but to find yourself and realize your powers, with nothing but the land. Absolutely no use of technology, no social media, no world news. Only your thoughts keep you company until your power is discovered and spiritually obtained.

I'm not talking about a few days like we see on the Discovery Channel, with a film crew and a helicopter nearby to bail you out if you decide you can't hack it. You have taken on this quest that may last months, and only you can fend for yourself. Do or die!

Now I realize many of us have not had or even been called to do this. Instead, the universe hands us another way to emerge into an awakening of ourselves with some of the greatest tribulations you can ever imagine.

Darkness and an abyss of nothingness are at your back and scorching hellfire at your front. There is nowhere to turn and nowhere to run. It's clear that nobody is coming to save you, and you feel more alone than you have ever felt in this life. There will be nothing glorious about this path you are about to embark on. No songs will be sung or poetic lines shall be written about your struggle. You close your eyes and wish it was nothing more than a bad dream. You hope and pray this struggle will quickly pass.

Your mind will do everything it can to find a way out of this nightmare, but no matter how hard you try, you're stuck. It becomes very apparent this has become your claim, this is your fight, and there will be no greater opportunity to grow and level up in your life than what you have right here, right now.

Solitude and loneliness are something many of us shy away from. The thought of loneliness frightens us. Have you ever asked yourself why? Is it because you need to be always entertained no matter whose company you keep? Is it because you need constant validation and reassurance? Is it merely because you have no idea who the fuck you are and you're terrified of the unknown? Or is it maybe because you have so much unhealed pain within yourself the thought of being alone literally frightens you?

If we are ever to heal and find power within ourselves, we need to change the current narrative of fear and solitude immediately. It is only scary if we label it scary. It is only lonely if we label it lonely. Start charging the narrative with positive energy rather than negative, and then you will have an excellent opportunity to get out of your own way.

During my darkest year, I did everything I could to keep myself busy. I always called my friends to invite them to dinner or a movie. I'd be at the gym two or even three times a day even though my body was spent. I did all I could to occupy my time all for the sake of not suffering the burden of being alone. Unfortunately, more times than not, I was left alone to deal with nothing but my blinding darkness and deafening demons.

I would be lying to you if I told you some of these days were not difficult. The mind can create some pretty unimaginable stories, and we do an even better job of believing them.

This is where the opportunity of creation emerges. Remember, just because you may be suffering from darkness and confusion does not mean that you are associated with evil or dark forces. Darkness is the realm where light is created. Where you have confusion only brings opportunities for reinvention. Where you cannot see, lies the opportunity to search within and find your true divine self.

So this is the opportunity to outright change your perspective and your intention. When dealing with darkness and traumas for so long, we allow them to run us like a sim on a computer.

Feeling completely hopeless and misdirected, we never once give thought to how we can turn the tides and change direction of this boat we're in from this continuous spiral.

One day, you decide to stand alone and find true beauty and power within yourself. That day, you stop believing in the old fabricated stories and the impossible standards this world has made you feel you need to obtain. Fear becomes acknowledged but never reacted to, and it is then you find your real power and become the Power within you!

The goal was never to end up forever alone. It was to find *who* and *what* I was by being still, with nobody else to find comfort or solace other than myself.

If you can find power and comfort with who you are, you will find an incredible power in parenting, friendships, and work relationships. Because you discovered the one virtue that too many turn away from: oneness with yourself—the ultimate power of solitude and self-acknowledgment.

Feeling alone, we encounter some sort of inner strength. Unfortunately, this isn't always the case. The many of us who decide to find solitude also engage extreme coping mechanisms along the way. If you need to find something to either numb yourself or distract you from being alone, there is no work being done. You are merely trading one variable for another.

Overworking is one example. Some believe it is harmless because they are only bettering their career and keeping themselves productive. Others partake in using marijuana, believing they will reap health benefits by daily or hourly consumption, but they end up high all day, numbing themselves from their very own existence.

Then there is the gym. To avoid loneliness, people overwork an already exhausted body, channeling pain through iron steel. This was me. I pushed my body at times further than I should have.

Like cutting myself, over-exercising was my coping mechanism. It was how, once again, I tempered my pain. Although I exhausted it for the day, the demons were awake and ready at any second, never allowing me a reprieve from the day.

These are examples of harmful activities that take time away from your true self while being by yourself.

If you need to create a coping mechanism to try and do the work, you are only deceiving yourself.

To find power in oneness, one has to find peace in the silence of sitting alone. Listen to your heart, and although music can be most useful and even healing, we cannot always depend on it to dictate and run our feelings.

In the work, we must acknowledge and honor whatever emotions we feel and not always be swayed or even amplified by what music can direct.

Give credit and permission to the emotions you feel. If you are sad, sit and figure out why, if you do not already know.

If you are angry or triggered by waiting in line for coffee too long, chances are there is another reason behind those feelings.

To find time to be alone, you're allowing yourself to discover more than just one channel. You can dissect your feelings and emotions, and by doing so, you can better control your triggers and projections rather than lash out at others and have them pay for the shit going on in your head.

I personally found power and solitude in nature. I never took advantage of the giant mountains surrounding my valley. Before I knew it, I was hiking with my dog up unknown trails.

I would purposefully leave my phone in the car and detach myself from any and all communication whatsoever. I would usually wait until right before dusk before I began my trek up the mountainside. I did so to give myself a better chance at being alone.

The mountains had become my new comfort, my new refuge, and my safe haven.

It never mattered on the season. If I needed to disconnect, up to the mountain I went. Sometimes I would go up for hours with nothing but a water canteen and a hunter's knife.

Now I don't recommend everybody heading up the mountain alone right before dark, but as a six-foot-three-inch 220-pound black man with a 150-pound dog that looks like a black bear, I reasoned my biggest threat would be a mountain lion or Sasquatch. I found healing by detaching myself from my comfortable environment and going literally into nature and expanding my consciousness. This was something I never took advantage of before.

By sitting on the mountainside, conversing with myself, as well as my god, not only gave myself permission to heal but also to cry. I was able to do so unbridled on more than one occasion. There was no one around to hear me sob, and the stillness of the mountain gave me a sense of peace

I had never felt before. It was almost as though the mountain gave me permission to let go, which I knew I could not do in any other location.

I understand for many, especially for most men, letting go is a hard emotion to give in to.

From the ages of 12 to 34, I had not given myself permission to cry or attended to my feelings. Shame, guilt, resentment, rage, and confusion made me unattached from expressing my emotions.

Without allowing the power of tears, we cannot allow ourselves permission to heal. This is the beauty of sitting with ourselves and giving us permission to do so.

There may be times when we don't even know why we are crying, which is perfectly okay. Not all emotions will have a name or a label to them. The point is to give ourselves permission to express how we feel.

According to Dr. Judith Orloff in an article published in *Psychology Today*, "Emotional tears have special health benefits." Biochemist and "Tear Expert" Dr. William Frey from the Ramsey Medical Center in Minneapolis discovered that reflex tears are 98 percent water, whereas emotional tears contain stress hormones that are excreted from the body through crying. Additional studies also suggest that crying stimulates the production of endorphins, our body's natural pain killer and feel-good hormones. "Interestingly, humans are the only creatures known to shed emotional tears, though it's possible that elephants and gorillas do too. Crying makes us feel better, even when a problem persists. In addition to physical detoxification, emotional tears heal the heart. You don't want to hold tears back." (2010).

Unfortunately, our culture has taught us it is unmanly or even shameful to shed tears, even for women in some households. When in fact crying is one of the greatest gifts we can give ourselves to heal. Instead, far too many of us hold all that shit in so we can uphold some story or backward truth.

By denying our tears, we make ourselves ready to snap sharply in anger to anything that annoys us due to the pent-up emotions we have stuck inside of us.

Remember, not crying does not make you any more manly or womanly, stronger or alpha, but acknowledging your emotions and dealing with them accordingly, correcting whatever trajectory you may be on, is one of the most heroic things you can do.

Although women are more likely to acknowledge their emotions than men, sometimes women build a wall of emotional sovereignty to deter their tears. There is no shame in healing, but only glory, self-empowerment, and gaining a knowledge of understanding that before was a heavy load.

Stop holding back your tears when you feel they need to be released. Stop hiding behind a story of embarrassment or dishonor.

These are only false stories and programs, making you feel crying is not appropriate nor accepted in our society, but in reality, this is a lie you have chosen to believe.

The avenues for healing are many, but the consistency of the work is, and always will be, yours.

Do not allow your healing to become just another coping mechanism of distraction.

Throughout this path of healing, I have seen many companions become obsessed with the work of self-healing, actualization, and betterment.

They listen to every podcast or audiobook possible. They love and connect with whatever is being taught. As they listen and learn, they think about who they can help and uplift with their new vast knowledge. Meanwhile, they never once apply anything they have learned to themselves and their path of potential rejuvenation. They become obsessed with the work without doing the work.

It is like a personal trainer who can explain every muscle, joint, and workout to better their clients, but is still heavily overweight because they have not applied their very own concepts of which they are mandating.

You can search outwardly day in and day out, looking for any help or a new direction to get you to where you want and need to go, but the truth for which you seek has always been deep inside of you.

As you begin this journey, you must be okay with being selfish with your time and your energy, which needs to be spent on YOU!

For parents, I know this is an overwhelming and somewhat unreasonable concept, but if you have no time because of the time dedicated to your children, you must find a way to make time. I realize this is not necessarily a solution but merely a fact.

I do believe the universe has a fantastic way of opening doors and opportunities when one decides to do this work, even if they cannot be seen immediately.

Remember, you are the sole creator of all your limitations. If you come to the foregone conclusion no time can be made, then no time will manifest. Change the narrative of your story, and you will then see your story be changed.

Be ever conscious of who you are spending your time around when you are back to your everyday reality. Are these people you are currently associating yourself with uplifting you in regard to your healing process? Or are they draining, negative, and not necessarily on the same road you are? It is essential to evaluate which energies you are allowing around you on this delicate path.

As you go through this process, take time to assemble essential warriors alongside you as you create your tribe. Find people who are on the same upward path as you are or who have been through this fight once before. Look to the knowledge, find new perspectives, and always listen and feel their story.

Do not be dismayed as some friends and family members go wayward from your circle for a while. Love and care for them still. Have faith and understand they may not support you in the way you may need, and you may not help them on their life course.

As you continue the work, small pieces will fall out or away, and stronger, larger pieces will replace that which was lost. As you build yourself, the proper tribe will begin to assemble around you as needed.

Rid yourself of the stigma that being alone is anything but your greatest opportunity to realize empowerment. No longer seek refuge in others or in coping mechanisms to avoid your real purpose and identity.

Always honor your feelings as well as your process, but be wary of becoming a recluse and avoiding the world and society altogether.

You have been called to this work to help those all around you, once you understand the grand capacity of power you carry.

Do not deny others the opportunity to hear your story or feel your strength. For you and only you could be the very vessel for one other person to have their eyes and heart opened to begin their work.

There are countless people every day beginning their solitary walk and finding their power for the first time, or once again.

As we commence, we all feel frightened, unsure, and question whether it is even worth it, but we begin the journey, nonetheless. It is okay to feel as you do right now. It's okay not to see the light at the end of the tunnel. Because in reality, there is no light at the end. You stepping up so courageously is the illumination.

Although physically, you may feel alone. Rest assured, we are many, seeking to find divine goodness within ourselves.

Allow the process to take its course. Wake up with intention each day and do the work.

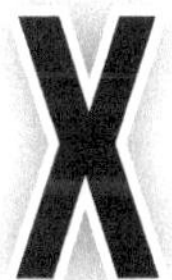

"As long as poverty, injustice, and gross inequality
persist in our world, none of us can truly rest."
Nelson Mandela

In 1999, I began my senior year of high school and had my first and only altercation with a police officer.

I was part of the top football team in the state of Utah, and we were about to reopen a crosstown rivalry with a team we hadn't played in the last few years. The timing couldn't be better. We were scheduled to play the team that continually whooped us all through Little League for the season opener on their turf.

This rivalry was just like every crosstown rivalry: full of bad blood and animosity. Our run-ins were probably much more subdued than what others may have experienced, and someone on the team usually had an adversary, a name, someone they despised greatly for no reason other than wearing a different jersey than we did, and perhaps for standing out on their team.

I felt our situation wasn't any different until a certain line was crossed. Not only was I challenged to fight a member of our rival team at the upcoming basketball game between our two schools, but he wanted to make sure that he told everybody he called me, "Nigger!"

So here we are again. First time since elementary, I was called nigger outright. So I was ready! I was angry and upset! Not to mention, I had my whole team as hype men planning for the Friday-night fight.

In actuality, after my nerves calmed, I wasn't ready. I wasn't a fighter.

I needed to have a breakout season that year to earn a scholarship. I was sad, scared, and dreading the day to come. Before the game started, not only did students from both schools know about it but so did the schools' administration and local police force.

As soon as I walked in the school with my entourage of teammates, I was quickly escorted to the principal's office with the other kid, and he ordered us to squash our plan to fight immediately, or we would both be suspended and kicked off our football teams. Even though I sat in my seat stoically, I was utterly relieved. I had no desire to fight. Although, I was greatly angered by another ignorantly charged comment. Still, I was never one to come to a violent resolution.

After the game ended, students from both opposing schools gathered on each end of the parking lot, barking choice words at each other, and before I knew it, we were surrounded by police officers, and I was handcuffed and bent over the hood of a police car.

Was I guilty of talking shit to the other school? Absolutely! But no more than anyone else.

As he had me on the hood of his police car, the officer threatened me, "I will throw your ass in jail so quickly, we don't put up with your kind!" I didn't respond. I was so embarrassed and ashamed as my friend's parents walked past me in disbelief.

I had never been in trouble before. I wasn't afraid of what was transpiring, I knew there was nothing they could do to me, but I wanted to crawl into a hole. My fear and constant insecurity were fitting the negative stereotype of a black man, coupled with already being a confused teenager.

After he ran my license and found there was nothing on me, he uncuffed me. I knew they already knew who I was, and they wanted to make an example of me, which they obviously did.

I took a few steps and then turned right back around and walked right back towards the officer. He quickly put his hand on his holster and urgently demanded, "Be Careful!"

I held out my hand, waited for what seemed like an eternity until he reached out his, dumbfounded. I shook his hand and said, "I'm sorry." As I turned around, my teammates looked just as confused as the officer. They asked why I did that, and I simply exclaimed, "I wanted him to know who I was." Which I did, not how he expected me to be.

I feel like I have been fighting bigotry my entire life. Sometimes through real-life scenarios like this exact situation, and others through the fabricated stories I decided to believe in to justify my paranoia.

The next day I was immediately called into the principal's office at my school, with the vice-principal, and our school police officer who held me in high regard.

As I walked to the table, to my surprise, they were more fired up than I was. They all wanted me to press charges. To be honest, their reaction caught me off guard. I thought I was about to be punished for the incident.

I reluctantly declined the opportunity to press charges against the officer. I didn't want to deal with the drama and distractions I knew would come along with it.

I sometimes reflect back on the altercation and wonder if I made the right decision. Should I have pressed charges to stop a potential Nazi with a badge? Or was it in my best interest to leave it as I did?

I share this to illustrate the inequality I have experienced, and not necessarily from police officers.

Throughout my career, I have worked and shared the rugby pitch and gridiron with many great officers of the law. I am still dear friends with many of them to this day.

I have experienced inequality and racial prejudice my entire life. So much so I began to believe I was lesser for the majority of my life.

It is incredible how easily we can believe in the lies our environment tells us.

I had always felt as though I was an alien: too black for the whites and way too white for the blacks. I never belonged to a tribe. I was simply a circle peg trying to fit into a square hole. I never fit, no matter how much I wanted to.

I felt like every minority or person of color had a tribe of the same kind to go home to, but not me, and this just added to the negative thinking I continued to pack away.

This just comes to show the power we have in our belief systems, and the power our belief systems have over us. We can believe in something so vehemently these convictions can lead to our very own betrayal if not unrooted correctly.

When racial injustices occurred throughout this country, I would feel more alone than ever. I had no one to lean on or share my concern or anger. I'd simply hear things like, "Well, if he wasn't breaking the law, he wouldn't have got shot!" Or, "Now that Obama is president, can we shut up about racism, please!?"

I am surrounded by many who have never even attempted to see the other side of the racial barrier because they have never had to. And like many, I would get heated over these politics and political feelings regularly.

After a while, I realized there was no use going into battle with those who did not share the same opinion. People are going to believe what they want to believe. Like all of us, we are going to try to believe what keeps us happy, which keeps us safe and sometimes even inflated.

We must remember, if you are to choose a stance or a side believing you are for the "greater good," equality and justice are not à la carte. You cannot accept certain justices and some equality and defer to other injustices and inequalities in the name of God, religion, or political affiliation. That is where I believe so many of us get lost.

Too many of us fear and shun away things we don't understand. We feel threatened by change and create a story that somehow, we'll be forced to acclimate to whatever "it" is.

We hear the phrase all too often now: *everybody is just so damn sensitive.* In some cases, this may be true. Is it also fair to say most everyone is in a constant search of just one thing? Being equal and fair. But what is equal and fair? What a subjective topic.

What I may believe is equal and fair to me may not be anything close to your core beliefs on this matter. As our positions become more and more fortified in this generational uproar, scathed with hate and non-bipartisan understanding, we feel our grip tightening as our message gets lost in this torrential downpour of other opinions.

Tradition and history have taught us there should always be one winner and many losers. One supreme and other subordinates. Man's quest for power and a fulfilled ego has tainted the balance of equality and corrupted the ability of self-love and understanding.

I also know and realize this sense of racial, religious, and political tyranny will forever be present. There will be the oppressors and those who are oppressed.

We can take this way of thinking all the way from world powers to the conformations in our own lives.

I have felt the nasty slap of injustice many times throughout my life and have tasted the bitterness and pain of inequality with barely anyone to empathize with.

My process of bearing this pain has been afflicted with loneliness.

Now without this chapter quickly turning into a political line drawn in the sand, leaving the feeling we all need to pick sides and take up arms, I simply want to share my personal observations and feelings of the manner I internalized those around me and basic core belief systems.

The results of a 2012 study by Stanford University found:

"A political science professor Shanto Iyengar and colleagues offers another way of looking at this apparent split. It examined political polarization from a different angle—not from how Americans stand on policy issues, but from the perspective of 'affect'—how they feel about those on the other side of the political fence. Drawing from survey data spanning several decades, the study found that the feelings of those who affiliate as Democrat or Republican towards members of the opposing party have become increasingly negative since the late '80s. The general pattern of dislike was mirrored by other specific metrics of 'social distance'— disapproval of one's child marrying someone from the opposing party as well as the attribution of negative stereotypes (e.g., close-minded, hypocritical, selfish, mean) to those of the opposing party, both of which have increased sharply since the '60s. Curiously, this 'affect polarization' wasn't so much related to ideology (i.e., where one stood on political issues) as much as partisan identity per se."

In a more recent study titled "Ideologues Without Issues: The Polarizing Consequences of Ideological Identities," University of Maryland Professor Lilliana Mason extended Iyengar's findings by distinguishing between two separate aspects of political ideology—"issue-based" (defined by what one believes about the issues) and "identity-based" (defined by one's social identity of party affiliation). In Dr. Mason's examination of political survey data, by far the more potent predictor of social distance was identity-based ideology—how we identify ourselves as Democrats or liberals as opposed to Republicans or conservatives—not where we stand on the issues.

Collectively, these results indicate that it's the social identifying role of ideological affiliation that's paramount in guiding our negative emotional responses to those on the other side of the political fence. This conclusion helps us to understand a few seemingly puzzling aspects of politics today—for example, how politicians can pivot on the issues when running for office and how key components of traditional party platforms can sometimes turn on a dime (e.g., the GOP and Russia) and why hypocrisy seems to run rampant in politics today.

For much of the voting public, political affiliation isn't so much about the issues as it is about being part of "Team Red" and "Team Blue." So opposed between "us" and "them," "liberals" become "libtards," "conservatives" become "fascists," and the possibility of finding common ground flies out the window. As NYU Philosophy Professor Kwame Anthony Appiah stated, "all politics is identity politics." According to these studies, it almost feels like we have become a nation of ride or die. We will defend our ideals, no matter where on the scale of morality they land. We will have a great distaste for the opposing parties and frame them in whichever negative manner we so choose.

Instead of coming upon a lifestyle, culture, or political beliefs with intent or searching for understanding, many instead apply the label immediately with fear and resentment simply because these beliefs or people are foreign.

It is time we are willing to work and change the narrative on how we are prepared to think about what is new and what is different.

Having friends I can sit down with and have entirely opposing political beliefs helps change the narrative around me. We talk and laugh with no ego and no intent to change the other's view. We bring our thoughts and ideas to the table in a very safe and secure manner. We both search for understanding rather than offense and ridicule.

Then we have those other friends and family members where we avoid those conversations altogether.

The quest to understand and discuss these touchy subjects should never be to dissuade someone from their beliefs but to understand. In return, it creates a higher gauge of understanding and intelligence for you and all who partake.

When was the last time someone yelled in your face or started a passionate battle with you on Facebook, and you were swayed away from your beliefs after a barrage of insults? Chances are never. Still so many choose to engage in this way of communication, feeling they are giving their beliefs validation. But let's be honest. It's your ego you are fulfilling.

How many friendships and family relationships have been ruined because of opposing views? You were both so passionate about how you felt, feelings were hurt, and in the end, both of you lost.

Please do not confuse intent on understanding with tolerance. We tolerate lousy weather; we tolerate a mean server at our favorite restaurant. Intent on understanding comes with looking at views from another perspective. Identifying that everybody has a different story than you and may come from a completely different culture and learning curriculum than you have.

It's time to put an end to our religious and political hierarchy. In many ways, these systems can make us better for our human experience, but not placing or esteeming us higher than the other.

I've seen so many people desperately and ferociously cling to the religious and political beliefs they have and never even give a thought to identify who they are as a person. Their beliefs in these systems are who they are, with no allowance of any other thought or opinions.

Like I said before, believe in what makes you happy but not to a point you are running a program day in and day out without any awareness of the power within you.

We are continually searching and seeking how to better ourselves via self-help books, enlightened conversations, YouTube, or whatever lights your fire, but what we forget is that the solution and direction are inside each one of us already. That awkward conversation many of us have avoided for so long.

David Goggins said it best, "We need to look inside ourselves." Stop running the program of the environment or culture you grew up in while being blind and cut off to what has been created already within you.

Like I had to learn the hard way, you are not meant to be like everybody else! You need to live for yourself first before you can live for anybody else. Learn to take pride in who you are and the way you think, rather than the shame and guilt this world has placed upon you.

Your unfulfillment and confusion come from external searching and validation. It is time to change your loyalty to your current belief system.

First, look inside and recognize the harsh judgments you carry towards others. Then recognize the fears that are influencing these judgements.

The Joker from *The Dark Knight* said, "Nobody panics when things go according to plan," but we panic when anything questions or challenges our belief systems. So we push back any sort of resistance with more resistance. Two opposing sides collide and never find a place of understanding and resolve. It is only through opposition we are given the opportunity for growth. Just as we build muscles in the physical body, we must allow for bedlam for mental and emotional growth.

Stop running away from uncomfortable conversations, but also learn to come to a place of allowance when opposing beliefs no longer trigger or threaten your ego.

What a power it is to control your own emotions and no longer allow others to dictate your reactions, no matter the situation.

The longer you decide to allow ego, judgment, and fear dictate who you are as a person, the longer you choose to inhibit your potential internal growth. You find no great purpose by avoiding that which is different from you, but only the opportunity.

I am not saying you have to agree or accept anything that is not in line with your core beliefs but simply eliminate your judgments led by fear. Take time to learn what you are afraid of or do not yet understand, and it will open you to a higher consciousness of understanding, patience, and resolve.

If we choose to stay in an immovable cycle, this cycle will only be perpetuated with a minimal awareness. Allow yourself to move in a way of thinking you may never have before. Give trepidation and guilt permission to leave, for they have never served you.

Some would say one can read and study all they want to become better and more enlightened, but if you continue on the path littered with judgment and egotistical sentiments, you are only crippling any chance of more significant growth, thereby dismissing the opportunity and power you have been given.

Now is the time to reevaluate your circle and your environment. Do all of your cohorts and work associates carry the exact same religious and political beliefs you do? Are the majority your associates all on the same page? Is the only place you differ in opinion the loyalty to your sports teams? If so, how is this environment serving you?

If you live life in a tunnel, with only limited vision for you to see, how can one grow? How can you be challenged?

Comfort is what cripples many of us from expanding our minds to higher learning and growth. The status quo is never challenged, even though we feel opposed to certain beliefs or sentiments of the majority. Most would rather keep their head down and remain silent and agreeable rather than speak the truth of justice and equality.

It is here failure is inherited. Not by loss, but by lack of voice, lack of truth, and lack of action predicated upon those truths.

To be "a product of your environment" doesn't always come with a positive connotation, and more so gives way to guilt by association, depending on majority views.

The great ones we look up to, in all walks of life, were never quiet and never normalized to the agreeance of their surroundings. Rather their voice was moved into action on a God-driven consistency until their dream and their calling became a reality for all to see.

Chances are, the ones you may look up to the most remind you of nobody else. Why? Because they have found their sole purpose and have fully stepped into their power. While so many others dream of shining out but are plagued by fear of rejection or exile that may come with their voice.

Many of us are in search of a higher power of goodness inside us and around us, but if you esteem yourself higher, better, or superior to another based on political, racial, or religious views, you have intentionally blocked yourself from finding the higher power and consciousness within you simply to feed an ideal(s) that supports a story that never has or will never be true. Feeding an ego with a foundation built on sand and fears.

For those of you who live by this theory, simply ask yourself to identify why these beliefs are within you. Are they of you, or were they implanted long ago? Do these belief systems bring you joy? Do they make your life better? Do they bring you peace? Be honest with yourself in this self-discovery.

Our world is plagued with followers, lemmings, and sheep. We need more lions, matriarchs, leaders, trailblazers, light seekers, and creators.

Step away from justified ignorance and its hooks that keep you no more than a puppet, playing along to the beat of an artificial drum.

If your beliefs allow you to place yourself higher than any one person, culture, sex, or sexuality, then it is time to not only question but challenge your credence entirely.

We do not need more bullies, but those strong enough to extinguish them by their effective affirmative action or silent, humble example. Refrain from using hollow words, which will disappear with no echo to follow.

Choose to seek and find your own path, discover the bright light within you. Fear only to remain the same, with a silent voice, while your heart not only cries to be heard but to also to be seen.

Open your heart to seeing truth and beauty in all things, people, and cultures.

Stop labeling judgments and fears on what you may not understand or have ever become accustomed to.

If you have the means to travel, then do so as often as you can. Engulf yourself with the people in new foreign lands. Ask questions, share stories, and most of all, listen! Pay attention to the sounds all around you. Listen to the tone of their voice as they share their stories.

What you will find is these people are not so different than you. Commonalities, laughter, and a connection will all be shared if you are only open to it.

If travel does not suit you, then do so in your hometown. The point is to see truths other than what you may have perceived as the one and only.

Remove the blinders of narrow mindedness and give yourself permission to explore more than the world you know today.

It is one thing to be corrected when we're unknowingly wrong, and another when we're able to emerge with realization, and we can obtain a new corrected truth.

As much as we'd like to give credit to our beliefs and current direction, we must exemplify understanding and openness that at times may very well oppose the belief system we clung on to for so long.

To move from long-standing beliefs can sometimes be very humbling and angering. Especially if one has felt hoodwinked by where we've formerly given homage.

To entirely remove oneself from what was thought to be true and move in a better, more precise direction is the truth of power to yourself. Give room and space to more truths that await you. This is an awakening!

Be that of resilient action. First with yourself, then with your household. Then you will see the true reach of your power.

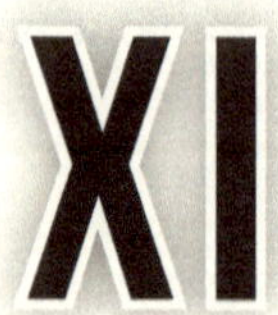

"Not to be cheered by praise, not to be grieved by blame,
but to know thoroughly one's own virtues and powers
are the characteristics of an excellent man."
Satchel Paige

I look back on my life with gratitude and a very scarred heart. There are so many things I wanted, and I really felt I needed, but those things were never given to me. By chance, I absolutely failed in my attempt to grasp them.

I just wanted a simple life.

There were so many times I wished I wanted to be a fireman, a lawyer, an accountant, or a successful sales representative with a lovely house and beautiful kids to raise. I fantasized about the mundane things my friends would complain about. I never once thought in my mid-30s I would be so broke I was forced to live at home with my dad because of my failed startup. I was barely able to make all my payments on time while still working ten-hour days.

Being broke kept me depressed for so long. In 2017, I applied for more than 1,500 jobs and was called for one interview. No matter how much I wanted to fit in, I couldn't. Even when I tried to force it, I would just get spat back out with the remembrance of not belonging.

I would beg and plead to God with tears flowing from my eyes, asking for financial help. I wanted to be an independent man once again so I could provide a beautiful home for my daughter, and most of all, finally buy a ring fitting for the woman I so dearly love.

I never pleaded for riches or glamorous things but to simply be sustainable once again and not miss meals because I had no money—or to borrow money from friends just so I could make all my payments on time.

It felt as though I was broke for years, and I never felt as though I would climb out of that hole no matter how hard I tried.

The first time I experienced being without, other than being a newborn, was my sophomore year of high school.

It was three weeks before Christmas when my family and I lived in a nice suburban neighborhood. My mother called me crying and screaming, "You need to get home Now! We have lost the house! We have 24 hours to get everything out or else we can't get it back!"

I quickly called my friends and told them what was going on. They got there before I did.

There was a moving truck already there, and my entire family and a few friends did everything to scramble and put our things into trucks as fast as we could.

It was a cold and snowy night. I remember going into my mother's room as she was tearing her clothes off the hangers crying hysterically and sobbing, "I can't believe this happened to us. I don't know what we are going to do!"

I still remember that day and the days that followed. I remember it changed my look on Christmas forever. A holiday I once loved so deeply had become tainted with painful memories.

Since I was the only child still living in my house, I moved in with my oldest sister, who lived by my high school. My parents moved about 20 minutes away with my other sister.

When Christmas finally arrived, rather than being a time of celebration and family, it was a time of sorrow and dismay. Many tears were shed as though we had just lost someone tragically.

My parents and sisters did their best to make sure we all had a sufficient Christmas. For me, it wasn't about the presents, even though I know my parents felt guilty they couldn't do more. It was about losing our home, our one place we could go to feel safe. It was our sanctuary.

I never quite recovered from that experience, and I may be able to equate it to the financial hardships I've suffered deeply in my adulthood.

This illustrates how unresolved traumas can rewire our memory of a story we sometimes choose to believe, either positive or negative. It also shows we aren't always as complete as we would like to be. Despite writing this book, I'm still learning and growing as time goes on.

Whenever Christmas comes around, and I hear the music and see the decorations, I feel sick—and I feel guilty for feeling so sick about it. Something I loved so much has now turned into a season I hate most. And because of my attitude, I have appropriately been labeled "the Grinch" during this festive season.

This is currently something I'm working on, though I've made strides to heal. My daughter motivates me to become better. Sometimes I wonder why, out of all of my life's struggles, is this one a trigger for me.

Perhaps this Christmas story further perpetuated the belief system already churning within me that there was never enough for me, and I was never good enough for anything or anyone else. I exiled myself years ago on an island of inadequacy. In essence, what transpired showed further evidence for my confirmation bias, which continued for two more decades of negative personal manifestations.

I chose to believe what I wanted to believe. I decided to see only what I wanted to see. I bathed in the dark of scarcity and continually would manifest meager monetary results.

As we search diligently to find our true selves and purpose, it is essential to identify those things anchoring us down.

The ever-present memories draw up so many feelings that we forget how to even function at times. The path to healing mentally and emotionally has been enormously more difficult than any physical challenge I had to overcome.

Some of us were never taught how to heal growing up, and self-healing sometimes comes to us at a crossroads, as it did for me. I could've pulled the trigger or made the absolute decision to heal. I took Andy Dufresne's advice from the movie *Shawshank Redemption*, "Get busy living or get busy dying." If you sit back and give time to think over your life and its mishaps, chances are you will find a common theme. Possibly the same anchor is still weighing you down today. Perhaps the broken heart you experienced more than once is from the same type of relationship you habitually create for yourself. Is this bad luck? Or is the dire lesson still waiting to be learned?

I believe the universe does a great job at manifesting the same lesson over and over again until the lesson is not only learned but also applied.

I do not believe tough lessons in each of our lifetimes occur on a linear pathway but rather on an elliptical one. In other words, the opportunity to learn and heal will present itself over and over again until the personal choice is made to accept the challenge of changing ourselves.

We have all seen the same situations, the same bad luck, the same type of toxic personality all showing up in our life. We wonder why we only attract a certain type of mate, or fall for the same deceptions, and ultimately ask, "Why does this always happen to me!?" Can you identify the common thread here? We see a consistency of situational patterns repeating themselves over and over, but instead of taking responsibility, we blame it on fate followed by #FML.

In "Invictus," Henley writes, "You are the master of your fate, and the captain of your soul!" Stop giving your power away by blaming external factors you fabricated in your head. If you have continual lousy luck, it's your fault! If you keep dating the same type of person and continually get broken-hearted, guess what? It is also your fault. If you keep losing money on the same desperate business investments? Guess what? It's your fucking fault!

The recurring patterns of disappointments are the lesson, not your luck.

Please read that again!

Do not keep forcing yourself into bad situations because your eyes and heart have not yet been opened. Do not be forced into healing because you are not willing to set your ego aside. When the universe has to force your hand, it can be worse than voluntarily doing the work.

Allow yourself to be broken down and created anew through this process. Continuously look for feedback from trusted sources, then integrate what you are being told. Before this counsel may have triggered your ego, but now it is received as invaluable information.

I now seek every opportunity I can for self-improvement, even when it stings a little. I then find gratitude in the changes people can openly see in me because of my work. Although, the point of this work is not to seek compliments or external validations. Compliments show us an external review on how others see our improvements and shift in energy.

An unhealed person with a huge ego will deflect away all criticism and help from those who love him most. Pride is his foremost motivator and drives away not only the counsel of others but those who so desperately care for him until he is all alone with nobody else left in his corner.

A humble and willing person will accept all counsel that is given, so they can be worthy once again for those who valiantly stand by him.

If you have multiple family members and or friends telling you the same words, encouraging you to get better, find help, or change in some way, it is probably time to pay attention to their message.

The counsel of angels can come from those dearest to us, and it doesn't always happen in some cinematic fashion in order to move us in a new direction.

Stop pushing away those who love you so dearly and want the best for you. It is time to step to the side and get the hell out of your own way!

Healing is not a get-rich-quick scheme. To find real success, you must put in the work. And there is no one right way to do it.

Depending on how deep your trauma goes, I always first recommend professional help. There isn't anything wrong with seeking professional mental help. For some, this is taboo. They believe it shows weakness or that something is wrong with you. That's not the case. Just like we must take care of our health physically, why are we not proud to share how we take care of ourselves mentally. People can be so quick to shout out and share their fucking workout of the day, but when it comes to strengthening our mental health, they're ashamed!

The old stigma of caring for your mental health is over. Mental illness has become an epidemic. Those too proud to go to therapy feed their ego and temper their pain with alcohol, drugs, sex, porn, gambling, etc.

If this is you, ask yourself, how is this really working out for you? There is nothing wrong with deciding to make yourself uncomfortable. Maybe for the first time ever, try to step out of your comfort bubble. Because really, that's all healing is. It's fucking painful and even scary at times, but it is far better than being stuck in a constant loop and playing chicken with endless blame and victimization.

As long as you continue to carry the shackles of trauma and pain, you will continue to thwart your entire progression in this lifetime.

In the words of Lewis Howes, "It is time to remove your mask."

Whether it's a mask of ego, comedy, submissiveness, pain, rage, or whichever mask you are clinging to, it is time.

It's ok to relieve yourself of your addiction to pain. I clung to it as long as I could. It was a part of me just as much as my limbs are attached to my body. Who would I be without my pain? What would there be left for me to hide behind? I needed my pain; I needed my rage, just as much as I needed air to fill my lungs.

In essence, removing that facade is literally removing part of yourself. It can be intimidating because the part of the unknown comes into play, but I promise you, the moment you decide to do so, your life will change forever. Your energy will begin to shift, and your outlook will start to change. Your triggers won't be so damn triggering, and most of all, your past will no longer dictate your future. Do not be afraid of the work! Be fearful of dying slowly from your past while you're still alive.

Not too long ago, I was recently told no matter what I did, as long as I didn't act myself, people would like me more. I didn't know how to respond at first, and ultimately, I didn't respond at all. It came at a time when I felt I had come so far to be who I was becoming. I didn't carry my wounds like a suit of armor anymore. I simply let my light shine forth.

What I realized is not everybody had recognized the new me. My past had given me a very unpopular image that still follows me around. Even though the real me was finally being uncovered, the old me was still an unsightly stain upon my character.

To move forward with this process, I could not throw away who I was before, only embrace who I was becoming. I had to love and accept all of me. If it wasn't for my darkness, my turmoil, and my traumas, the man I only thought was a figment of my imagination would not be forged into the all-powerful man I am becoming.

Self-hate, regret, and shame of who you once were sheds nothing but produces unruly conflict to who you really are. No matter what laid the foundation of your past, it brought you to this very moment of opportunity to finally emerge recreated as the person you want to be.

Whether your past hardships are the fault of yours or others, the point stays very much the same. Remember how I explained blame? Same concept. It still doesn't change your current situation once the blame is issued. Find a way to become grateful for who you are now, shedding off what is old to grow anew.

The goal of life is not to be perfect and without scars, marks, or embarrassment, but to simply correct your trajectory from where you thought you were supposed to be going. The ability of recognition, accountability, and recourse.

For many of us, self-examination is ongoing. For those of us practicing self-examination, we constantly ask ourselves, "Am I good enough? Am I worthy enough? Am I loved? Am I wanted? What do I have to offer?"

If we allow external factors to become way too involved in our own forward thinking, we may disregard our internal power because our power is something we cannot always see or feel. We move through life searching for evidence of our self-worth rather than creating what is already ours.

As I did my dance with darkness, I deeply questioned my existence as a man. I too believed in the fabrications my mind created.

We are swayed to believe in such self-damaging lies if we do not grasp the power within us.

A few months after I set my gun down once and for all and continued to fight my demons, fears, and current financial situation, I began to realize how precious and sacred my life was. Contrary to the backward thinking that everyone else's life was more valuable than mine. I shudder to think how tragic it would have been if I pulled the trigger—the experiences I would have missed and the invaluable growth I would've dispensed of.

I began to look at my life in a whole different light. I appreciated the man I became physically. I worked out to improve who I was, not to inflict punishment. I was able to acknowledge my growth intellectually as I became obsessed with the search for new knowledge calling out to me. I was able to create a space of self-love and appreciation I never once knew before.

My focus shifted, and although there still would be bad and dark days, they occurred less and less, and then the not so bad days became more prevalent. Soon, the I'm-happy-I-am-alive days outnumbered the bad.

Understanding this was mine and my own responsibility specific to me was hard but a very liberating lesson to apply to my life. I alleviated my mind of any notion I needed saving in one way or another, and if I simply waited out the storm, everything would just get better. The moment you can rid yourself of the fallacy that you are a victim, and you will somehow be saved is when divine power begins to grow within you.

Gaining a new perspective creates an opportunity to become much more self-aware. You are cognizant of your triggers and find a line back to why they are even triggers. You can better understand why you are the way you are.

How can you know or even be aware of your shit until it's identified?

It took me the majority of my life to realize the innate spiritual beauty I hold. I spent my years concentrating on what had been taken, forcing energy into what I felt and the lack thereof. When in all reality, I was looking out the wrong window. It took me forever to understand positivity and manifestations are great and mighty things because I had been so obsessed with the dismay of all my experiences.

You have the power to choose which window you would like to look out of in this life. Even when bad things happen, we can bring ourselves back to beauty. We can no longer submit to pain as our master. Just as I can no longer allow the memory of an eviction to taint so many wonderful opportunities to recreate what I once loved so very much.

I allowed my pain to manifest over and over again for more than 15 years. And with that, I relived the very same Christmas each year, and many of those years, I was alone. Manifesting what I hated so much, I did not have the wisdom to shift from my current state of blame.

Be willing to break your ongoing cycles of pain. Come up with a new plan, and if the plan doesn't work, be willing to pivot again until one does.

I have wasted so many experiences because of my choice to succumb to sadness. I simply was not aware there is another way to look into my past, so I could be powerfully present right here and now.

Nothing will ever magically get better. You will not one day suddenly wake up healed from your past. Just like you will not magically awake with a new talent, skill, or extraordinary power.

This art of healing is earned, level upon level. With each new power attained comes a price. Which is the emotional and mental anguish you allow yourself to let go of finally takes diligence and much courage. This is the work of a Warrior. This is why many will not answer the call and instead continue life sinking in quicksand and resulting in minimal growth.

Come to terms with who you are meant to be. You no longer need to be where you are or where you have been. There is no greater feeling once this concept is brought into your every waking reality.

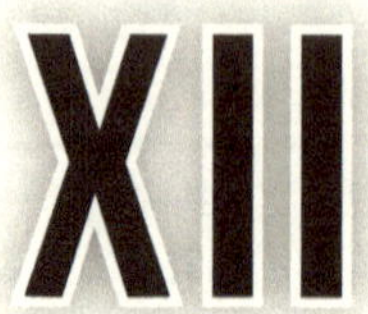

*"Hatred and bitterness and anger only consume the vessel
that contains them. It doesn't hurt another soul."*
Rubin Carter

To some, my story may seem pretty significant, and to others, it may seem to be a simple life compared to what they've gone through. Although I was left in this life with so many unanswered questions, over time, I allowed space to answer them the best I could. Through this journey, I was given many options and opportunities to not only let my pain and anger define me but become me. All of us have or will experience darkness to some extent. What is important is that we do not feel it necessary to compare our darkness to the likes of another. Dark is dark. We all have the ability to deal with it differently.

I wondered if it were possible to yield to the evil of the darkness in my state of confusion. I considered to go out and seek revenge to all who betrayed me, to act out in vengeance to this unfair and unbalanced world. Although I had flirted with the notion, I would merely be reciprocating the same deeds that were done so unjustly against me. I toyed with these thoughts amid my confusions and dreary days, but I never once became them, and they never became of me.

Do not confuse imperfections with the intent of wrongdoing or horrible acts.

Our stories usually make us one of three people:

The first person we become is more empathetic and patient with the world. Our heart opens to the sad and troubled. We offer help where we can because we are the ones who understand what it is like to go through tumultuous pain and agonies of defeat. Therefore, we become more constant for those who share the same road we once or still are trudging against.

The second is numb, apathetic, and completely unattached. These people have disconnected themselves because of the horrible traumas they experienced. They willingly or unwillingly chose to go on through this life with no more emotional feeling. These are those who have no power because they have chosen to accept no control, and they blow along in this life like a leaf in the wind.

The third type of person has chosen to become the bad, the angry, and overtaken by the very rage they once experienced. This type of person has chosen to allow others to experience the same pain they experienced. They seek revenge on a pain that can never be brought to justice.

We see these people day in and day out with the awful whoredoms advertised on every news channel. For most of us, we cannot understand how someone is capable of committing such atrocities. But unfortunately, they happen every day, and the violence only seems to get worse and more frequent.

How many times have you seen hate or malice in someone's eyes? Other than television, I can only account for a couple of times, and each was racially motivated.

My family had moved into a new neighborhood, and I was to start kindergarten. We lived only a few blocks from the school, so my sister and I walked together every day even though we did not get along. She would usually take off in front of me and catch up to a girlfriend or two, and I'd trail behind. I often got distracted by whatever bugs or wildlife I could find along the trail to school.

On one particular day, there was a group of teenagers walking in my direction. At such a young age, our minds do a grand job of exaggerating our reality, and they seemed much older and larger than they were.

As I walked through them, one of them threw me to the ground and yelled, "NIGGER!" They all walked off laughing as they continued on their way. I laid on the ground in confusion, not only for being thrown to the ground but for trying to understand what the word nigger even meant. I had never heard it before.

I picked myself up and continued to school as though nothing had happened, saying nothing to anyone about it.

The next few days, I was definitely apprehensive about walking to school again.

A few weeks went by, and I hoped that event was just a one-time occurrence. But there they all were, once again, a human roadblock on my way to school.

Did I run? Hide in the bushes? I walked on hoping they didn't notice me. My intention was not to be tough. I was like a deer frozen in headlights and had no idea where else to turn. I looked up and down the street, praying to find an adult outside their house, but to no avail.

As soon as the teenagers saw me, they looked at each other and started laughing and quickened their pace. I don't recall how many there were. All I remember is that before I knew it, I was back on the ground and hearing the word "NIGGER" over and over again from each of them.

This time they didn't keep walking. I began to feel a barrage of kicks and fists all over my body. I tried to get up, but the assault continued to rain in.

The memory of white Converse PF Flyers one of the kids was wearing. After the beating was over, the kid wearing the Flyers bent over while I was still on the ground, and it was there I saw it for the first time . . . sheer hatred!

He looked right at me and said, "You nigger!" As spit flung from his lips and onto my face. To this day, I still can feel precisely where every drop of his saliva stained my face.

When they felt satisfied after what seemed like an eternity, they scampered off, laughing the whole way. I remember getting up and seeing an older woman with a broom, standing in her driveway where it all happened. She looked concerned but never said a word. I looked at the damage over my body. It wasn't nearly as severe as I was scared. I had a few bumps on my head, but most of the scrapes were from the asphalt.

I remember walking into school right after the bell rang, and my teacher asked why I was late. I said I fell while running on my way to school. I never said a word of what happened that day until much later in my life.

I ran into the boys a few more times, but I decided to be smarter. I would run and hide. Until one time, my sister saw what was happening and told my parents. I never had to deal with them again. Although I ran into a couple of them at church on Sundays, no words were ever said. Just a few laughs amongst themselves when they walked by.

I never really had anyone to turn to when I faced bigotry. I had no one who really understood or who I could relate to.

As I look back, I find a greater feeling of gratitude for my parents and siblings. Even though they could never quite empathize with what I was going through, it didn't matter because they had my back and were always there to protect me.

I can only imagine the consequences I may have suffered if I didn't have a safe place to go home to with the love and support I received.

However, I did realize that not having anyone to relate to caused me to repeat the same cycle through my elementary years. I was bullied significantly through seventh grade. During that time, I would find other kids to pick on. Since it was happening to me, why couldn't I do the same and be justified in perpetuating the cycle?

Luckily for my very aware father, I was put in check really fast. My attempts to balance things out in my eyes were put to an immediate stop.

This vicious cycle is precisely how it starts. The abused becomes the abuser. Revenge and vengeance are sought upon by the once victims. To fill or justify the very sins committed against them. And depending on the significance of the wound amplifies the desire to inflict on another. And sometimes to horrifying consequences.

We as parents need to become more aware of the cycles we pass on to the vibrant sponges we call our children. The negative cycles must end with us, or else we may suffer unimaginable consequences.

We must also realize, no matter what has been done to us, we are always still left with a choice. We all know one person who has been through some of the most horrific events in life, and yet they are still the softest, most loving human beings imaginable. They know all too much what hell looks and feels like, and they would do anything to make sure they can help anyone to avoid any sentiment of it if they can.

Then there are those who we know and see who have become the very thing they have come to hate. They stop at nothing to project their pain on anyone they come in contact with, either through energy, verbal abuse, or violence.

Their minds have become fixated on revenge and self-gluttony. They aim to make others feel what they feel, to make others pay for the way they have paid. It is a sad reality many of us have seen and experienced because the cycle of trauma continues on to another and another.

I have seen too many become perpetrators of the abuse and ridicule they once experienced. With an inflated ego of entitlement, they press others to subjugation and intimidation to ultimately become victims to live through the very same experiences they once did.

Unwilling to move nor to see, they are casting the very same stone, only to a different lot. These cycles must be decimated from a very aware and willing soul to do the work. So how does one who is blind accept the responsibility to step away from their plaguing projective habits? Unfortunately, there is no single antidote for those suffering under the tyrant of such abuse.

In Charles Dickens' *A Christmas Story*, we are told of the ill-favored character Mr. Scrooge who throws down his cane of pain and oppression all around him. None were free of his misery's path. All until he was visited by three ghosts on Christmas Eve to help him realize his shocking ways and allow him to correct himself. This may be farfetched for some, but still a very excellent example of how cycles are perpetuated.

How many times have you found yourself on such an egotistical or self-righteous path, and life put you in a situation where you had no choice but to correct it? Life has a funny way of redirecting our course even if it is not asked for.

I do believe those who continue to act recklessly with their power and authority are given opportunities to redirect their path but won't take the bait. We may wish they receive their comeuppance soon, but what an even greater waste of energy we expend by harboring those feelings.

The feeling of witnessing men like this fall is never what I imagined it to be. Rather than celebration and joy in my heart, I experienced frustration and felt sadness for them because they never took the time to see their missteps and to allow their heart to heal; karma not only tripped them up, but it slammed them with a Mac truck.

I knew of a man with a very similar story and background to mine.

He grew up a minority in white suburbia and faced the same trials and rejection as I did. He never knew his father until he was older, and his mother suffered from her own demons, causing the cycle of trauma to continue and pass along to him.

This man was able to find his success, find his calling, and find his path. He shined in ways I could only dream of. But even with all his success and dreams achieved, he never gave a chance to put his own demons to rest. Instead, they led him. He became self-justified in his tyrannous actions and oppression towards others. Like a loose cannon, he'd fire at anyone in his way, consequently losing his marriage, his family who took him in, and a long line of friends, one by one. Finally, the process of losing his children began. They were no longer willing to accept the abuse and ridicule, which was once passed along tragically to him.

He was traumatized by abandonment, and he witnessed horrible things as a child. Unfortunately, he carved out his path with no apologies and egotistically excused his own actions.

I believe he subconsciously expects everyone will eventually leave him, like he was left as a small child. Although hugely successful, he never moved out of survival mode. He sacrificed relationships just to keep a standard of living and a name for himself. His pain blinded him of the things most valuable in this life, and his ego and stance remain strong and will remain strong to the point of self-exile unless he finds a way to see himself and how his actions left a trail of bodies and lost relationships littered along his path.

Although his rage and pain propelled him forward in his career, he was never able to control how he filtered his sinful energy.

Attempting to manipulate our negative energy becomes such a slippery slope for many of us who have seen more days that are worse than better. Our heart is another empty black hole filled with acts of corruption, rage, and despair. Sometimes one's heart cannot become anymore broken, and then the decision is made. Their path is the path where pain and dark energy are projected on innocent victims.

In my darkest of times, I never once thought to harm or cause pain to others, only to myself. But then again, my pain, my experiences were different. I can never stand here with judgment to those who have experienced such tragedies that their lives will never be the same. My heart breaks for them and all who suffer so deeply.

How great are those who experienced unimaginable travesties and still choose to do the work! They decide not to exact their revenge. The cycle ends with them, and a new, more powerful, abundant cycle begins.

No matter what is experienced in this life, there is always a choice. As imperfect humans, we do not always make right or logical decisions. We do not always know how to react appropriately.

Turning the other cheek hasn't always been an option for me, and like you, there are certain extreme cases where you wouldn't either. We have to be able to own up to whatever consequences come after.

Rarely in this generation, and generations before, has much been accomplished without intelligent resistance. Make no mistake, there are times to fight, there are times to overthrow, and there are times to resist.

But right here and right now, if you are to fight, fight back through your pain, through the limits and lies you've believed for so long! If you are going to overthrow, overthrow your belief system of egotism and revenge. Overthrow the feeling that your negative behavior is justified, and you are set higher among anyone else. And if you are to resist, resist the pitfalls of the same patterns and spirals that overwhelm you with hopelessness, and there is no point to continue on or even try.

There is always a choice; there is always a path. You are responsible for the conscious decisions you make in the here and now. Run away no longer from the hard or the uncomfortable choices. Lose the desire to follow the crowd or the majority. Do not limit your power nor potential of your true purpose out of fear or contentment.

For this is the fight of your life. Do not waste any longer on what was and give absolute power to what can be.

Take responsibility for your reactions in every situation. Power is having control over your emotional and mental responses. Become aware you may be walking a fine line between the projection of negative energy and protecting yourself. Or the realization you may have already taken a step into the very place you resented so severely. If you find yourself in that place, become accountable to make every possible change to move away from it altogether.

How often have you walked away from a situation embarrassed or ashamed of the way you reacted? Or come to a standstill, eyes locked on yourself in the mirror, wondering how the hell did you get to this place? We all have or soon will.

Our goal is to avoid that point altogether, where we feel we have fallen so far, we don't know how to climb back up.

After my divorce, I had an outside sales job that paid decently. I was living in my own place and completely independent. I had all my bills covered, and I was able to buy the things I needed. I was in completely the wrong space for the products I was selling, but I had been at this job for a little more than two years when I received my biggest commission check. This commission check was a game changer. I was able to qualify and buy my very first house. I was so proud of myself. I was excited for my daughter to have a place to call a place home.

I was very responsible for paying down all my accrued debt, and my credit score was well over 700.

Because of that, I planned to close on my loan and my house the very week I received a call from my boss stating he'd like to meet with me while he was in town. I thought he simply wanted to see how the territory was growing and meet with new and old sales opportunities. I set up meetings for the days he would be in town.

After the first day of meeting all of our current customers, we planned to meet the following morning at a local coffee house before we drove a few hours south to another potential client.

Arriving right on time, I found my boss seated at one of the booths with papers and his laptop. Before he moved to headquarters in another state, he managed my territory. He left behind his wife and kids because of a diminishing marriage.

"Sit down, Rob." From his tone, I knew what was happening.

I sat down. "Rob, we are going to have to go another direction. I, unfortunately, am going to need to move back home and take care of my family."

"I don't understand; I took this territory from last to first in less than a year."

"I understand that, but this is my call," he said.

"So I am losing my job because you are moving back?" I asked.

"It appears that way," he arrogantly replied.

"I am closing on my house this week. There is no way my loan will get approved once they find I am no longer employed!"

He shrugged at me with annoyance as to say, "So?"

He reached out his hand to shake, and I reluctantly grasped it. It took all my power not to pick his big ass up and body slam him on the table.

I drove away, absolutely bewildered. Like clockwork, driving home, I received a call from my loan office to notify me they could not find proof of employment, and for now, my loan would be placed on hold.

Just like that, I lost a job and my first house within minutes.

Four days later, I received the news that my best friend had taken his life, the brother of mine I had felt responsible for.

A week after that is when I discovered that the first girl I had given my heart to after my divorce was sleeping with everybody else but me.

And just three days after that, I had to put my dog of 13 years down.

I was fucking demolished!

A few days after everything transpired, I remember sitting under the clouds on my front porch after a long day. The gray sky quickly turned to what seemed like a monsoon. The hot summer air quickly turned to cold wind, and rain smacked my face with every forceful drop.

I didn't get up; I didn't run to shelter. I just sat there. This was a culmination of not only the worst three weeks of my life, or the worst month, but the worst time of my life altogether.

I was on what I thought the precipice of success and stability was only a few weeks ago. There I was, sitting in the rain, hoping to be blown away out of existence.

It was so hard to breathe as the summer storm blasted through me. I sat through the entire storm unaware if it lasted minutes or hours. I was numb and never more broken until right there at that moment.

All the pain we endure is calculated and quantified. If not addressed and dealt with, the traumatic three weeks I experienced is a perfect example of where your road may lead.

After I graduated high school, I moved to Hawaii on the North Shore with some of my close friends for a couple months before I started college. I fell in love with the land as well as the ocean.

One day, we went bodyboarding on a break we definitely were not experienced enough for called Log Cabins, but we continued anyways.

On my first attempt to charge a wave, I caught it too late and nosedived toward the ocean floor. Luckily, I missed the reef, but as I came up for air, another colossal wave toppled over me, pushing me down once again. I was caught in what's called the impact zone. This lasted for at least three more waves. Coming up to barely gasp for air and then being pushed back down again, I thought I most assuredly wasn't going to make it to the surface. It was terrifying.

After the set was done, I paddled with what little energy I had left to shore and sat the rest of the day out because of exhaustion and immense fear. On my first attempt, I got my ass kicked.

What an interesting foreshadowing of what would occur fifteen years later.

I got caught in the impact zone once again and couldn't breathe. When it was finally over, I did exactly what I did on the beach that day. I quit. I didn't move forward, didn't attempt to heal or resolve any of my decades of layered issues. I was just another victim with no sense of direction.

Although I felt terribly saddened, scared, lost, and betrayed by life, I never once wanted my pain to become an act of vengeance.

Even though so many close to me fell victim to my low and dark energy, I kept my integrity intact. For those negative thoughts have never been part of my character.

You never are to become a victim of your circumstances or how you choose to react because of these circumstances.

Find humility in your specific circumstance, but never react out of a dark heart with ill intent.

There is power found in the warrior who can stay his sword and not react out of blood lust cursing the world for his pain.

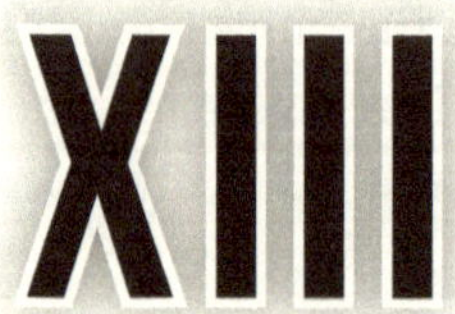

*"When you know who you are; when your mission is clear and you burn
with the inner fire of unbreakable will; no cold can touch your heart;
no deluge can dampen your purpose. You know that you are alive."*
Chief Seattle

One afternoon, I picked up my six-year-old daughter from kindergarten. As all loving fathers do, I dote on my daughter, telling her how beautiful she is and how much I love her. As she climbed into the car, I asked her, "Amari, why are you so beautiful and amazing?"

She contemplated the question for a moment and responded, "You know, Dad, I just know who I am."

Tears filled my eyes as I drove. I turned and looked at her. I had to see my daughter after that profound statement. No one had ever astounded me the way my six-year-old just did.

The fantastic thing about her statement is how she said it with both innocence and conviction. She knows who she is, and she loves it. This is the beginning of the Warrior: someone who knows who they are and loves themself. They understand their flaws and shortcomings, but they honor and amplify their strengths.

On the other hand, there are those who experienced much affliction in their life, beaten down by never-ending waves of disappointment and subdued by tireless beliefs of pessimistic thought, perpetuating the vicious cycle of victimization through their cursed words, jealousy, and hate.

Throughout my life, I was always looking for something or someone other than myself to blame. Even though not all the blame was mine, it still didn't change my situation. I was angry, I was lost, and I had always felt alone.

I had to come to a point where I eventually became obsessed with my frustrations of being unsuccessful and unfulfilled with my life.

I sat there and witnessed nearly all my friends have established careers, big houses, and a family to come home to. Here I was, 36 years old and dead-ass broke. I had taken some hits, some ass whoopings, and significant heartbreaks. I had become the poster boy for victimization. I had lost everything and was broke for what felt like an eternity.

In actuality, I never made much money, and to be honest, I had never been entirely responsible with it. I grew up seeing many around me leverage things they couldn't afford with credit cards and continue spending beyond their means. Unfortunately, I adopted that unfavorable way of thinking.

I am not upset with myself for investing more than twenty thousand dollars in a product I invented but never came to fruition.

However, I failed in a variety of areas that led me to that point. First, I somehow convinced myself since this life had dealt me so many bad hands, somehow someway the tides would change and miracles would start appearing before me.

What a trap I fell into. Fabricating remarkable stories of triumph and success with absolutely no work or dedication to my mental or emotional wellbeing.

Second, I created the most elaborate, tear-jerking success stories in my head, and I became enamored with what was just a fantasy rather than digging myself out of this enormous hole with progressive action.

Last, I became lazy. Not with my weekly work hours, but by working in a way I never had before. To get me out of the stagnant way of thinking to create results, I had for so long become a slave to my mind and my ego. I felt this world owed me, and my ego created the lavish luxury ride into the sunset dream.

I believed it would one day fall into my lap, but it never came to be. I remained broke for much longer than I ever should have.

I carried shame wherever I went, simply because I could not find my direction or sense of purpose.

Being an empath and overly sensitive has led me to a lot of wrong decisions throughout my life. I had been taken advantage of more times than I would like to admit by friends and business associates. I always tried to see the best in others, and I felt I knew they would be as loyal and forthright to me as I was to them. More times than not, those relationships never panned out.

I depended on people to provide more than just an idealistic friendship but my livelihood. In reality, they watched me sink with a smile on their face then turned their backs on me.

I was so desperate for acceptance and love, I assumed those I trusted would graciously meet my needs. To my dismay, they did not.

I created so many stories with my victim mentality. I needed so much external validation and success to know who I was.

Growing up, I always searched for a place of belonging, a family, a tribe. I knew I was different, and I was even ostracized through grammar school. I yearned to belong somewhere. Though I got a small taste of it through sports, especially in high school, I never really belonged, and it still feels true in many ways to this day. I don't have a culture or ancestral heritage to call my own.

I like to think I came from a great lineage of great kings and tribes of warriors who fought for good and righteous ways, but those are just daydreams.

I longed to belong to a culture of ancient traditions of great pride. I searched relentlessly to answer the question of who I am and where I come from, but each person I've hired came to a dead end.

I, in turn, created my own culture of what I wished and envisioned I came from. I researched West African symbolism, which helped me create the tribal tattoo along my left shoulder, back, and arm. Each symbol carries a sacred meaning and power specific to me and what I aspire to be. These markings give me a sense of hope and connection to a family and heritage I may never know for sure is mine.

Because of the unanswered questions, I had no choice but to dive deep within myself and my mind. I questioned who I was really and what my purpose is. I realized I didn't have to depend on stories or traditions written before me. I wasn't obligated to go down a path that didn't fit who I was. Even though I wish for the contrary, no greater force occurred to me than to answer these questions for myself.

Because I lacked the foundation of growing up without identifying and sharing commonalities with my peers, I was subjugated to a lot of self-doubts. I questioned everything I did. I could only fake self-confidence, when in reality, I had none. This hindered me immensely from obtaining my full potential in all my endeavors. I hid behind a façade of self-assurance, warding off anyone who dared come close to me.

Because of the community and religious culture I grew up in, I attached myself to a lot of guilt and shame. I felt guilty for not achieving and living the religious standards I was supposed to, and I felt shame for the mental and emotional anguish I inflicted upon myself.

Most of us who feel guilt or shame punish ourselves because somewhere in our head, we believe we deserve punishment for not being good enough. We abuse ourselves, and we become disloyal to ourselves, therefore manifesting other dysfunctions in our own reality like self-doubt and fear.

Self-doubt is the greatest dream killer known to man. Like cancer, these thoughts will eat at every potential creation one has formed, and before the idea can ever come to action, it has been killed off by the deadly disease.

In *Pirates of the Caribbean: World's End*, Jack Sparrow and his gang of pirates didn't exactly know how to escape Davy Jones's Locker. All they had was a map with the clue "Up is Down." They eventually figured out they needed to capsize the boat to magically reappear to reality as they knew it.

For me, the only way to make it out of my trauma and level up in this lifetime was to go down. To be brought to my knees, humbled, and then kicked down again.

Hitting rock bottom is terrifying because you can only think of when it will end. I begged and pleaded to be saved, but nobody ever came to save me. I didn't know my rock bottom would last as long as it did, and it lasted years.

I had to navigate myself out of this mess, and it was nobody's responsibility but my own to do so. I wanted to quit, I wanted to give up, and more than anything, I wanted to exist no longer. I was defeated, and in my heart of hearts, there was no more fight in me to give, no more reason to crack on. My only escape was the three to four hours of sleep I'd get a night. Then I'd wake up to live out the same waking nightmare all over again.

How did I get through it? I made a choice.

Here's an example that may help you gain perspective.

On the plains of the Midwest and through the Rocky Mountains, both cows and buffalo roam the vast lands. Although they are similar in size, their mental outlook is entirely different.

When a storm is approaching, the cows take notice and begin to head in the opposite direction of the storm. Obviously, never being able to outrun it, they do their very best to escape the inevitable.

On the other hand, you have the buffalo. When the storm rages toward them, they begin to charge at it. They have the mindset of taking on the challenge of the storm, willing to bear the winds, the cold, and the rain. They push through as fast and strong as they can until the storm is over.

You have a choice. You can run from what is, knowing it will continuously be there as it continues to rage on. Or you can turn and face the storm and take it on with all of your might!

A young man battling severe depression and suicidal thoughts was asked how he had persevered. He simply replied, "One more day." He continued to explain every day was hell for him, but he made a promise that if he made it through yesterday, he would make it through one more day.

He made a daily decision to carry on one more day.

Darkness and trauma are caused by significant events and heartbreak and can be medically diagnosed as you search endlessly to identify and cure your condition.

Remember, if you got through yesterday, you can get through one more day. I recommend you do it with intention. Set the intention to get better and not lie in your shit any longer. Set the intention to know you'll be able to deal with horrible days, and you will have days where you'll look back and see weren't quite so bad. Set the intention to have even better days. Intention is followed by action.

Tupac Shakur said, "After every dark night, there's a bright day after that. So stick your chest out, keep your head up, and handle it."

Specifically finding what works for you. Not what worked for them but for you! If you think back over your life and consider the people you have befriended, fallen in love with, the experiences you cherished, entertainment you indulge in, and routines you commit to, how much time have you taken to get to know you!? I bet not as much as you could have.

Have you searched deep inside yourself and given yourself the opportunity to fall in love with yourself? Or do you look in the mirror with displeasure and harsh critique? Have you based your success and purpose by comparison of social media pages because you've become so concerned by what "they" are doing, rather than investing in you?

If comparison is not your problem, then your task is to identify what your problem is.

The human heart is meant to be open and shared with the rest of the world. Our abundance resides when we share our stories, connect our souls, our strengths, as well as our faults with one another. Doing this will no longer give us the need to pretend to be something we are not, to no longer preach words as a disbeliever and non-compiler. Take note of our past and find what and why it makes sense to this present and future.

Find the power of standing and healing alone, but in no way feel you are too broken, sad, or lost to stay alone. Share your strength and your story with those who deserve to hear it, and maybe those who don't. Recognizing you are not alone in this mess called life is nothing short of amazing.

We all have a story, and more than likely, we have all been brought to our knees. Where we find strength is through the ability to find solace within ourselves, through ourselves, and become an extension and lend a helping hand to others in their new path.

Everybody manages pain differently and in the best way they know how. Most of us were never taught how to heal, how to operate, and how to move on. Remember, trauma forever changes the person we are today. But, we can choose who we want to become if we work at it.

Each great adversity in our life presents an opportunity for us to be more than the cliché of becoming better and stronger. This isn't always the case. Sometimes the lesson of adversity is to find out who we really are and what purpose we are meant to fulfill—to connect wholly with our soul, our hearts, our Warrior. This is the fight we have in this physical and spiritual form to find our true selves once again, even after all the shit and hardships this world has dealt us.

Life will continue on the same cycle, with the same lessons until the lessons are learned. Opportunities and experiences are not linear. If we believe in a higher purpose, then the greater purpose will present itself over and over until that purpose is fulfilled.

Once you set aside your ego, I mean really set it down, you will know what is holding you back from becoming the person you know deep inside you are supposed to be. You know where you are being lazy, fearful, egotistical, and unaware. The right path for you is waiting to be discovered, but only if you have the courage to uncover it.

During my path of discovery, I identified with the lion so much so, it is permanently marked on my back.

I had the opportunity to get up close with a lion a few years back with a VIP pass to a theme park.

This male lion, with a vast, beautiful mane, sat there peacefully but watched ever so carefully what I was doing. I walked right up to him, with only steel bars separating us. We were face to face and made eye contact. Something occurred that I had never experienced in my life. This lion not only didn't break eye contact, but his stare went straight through me. I can honestly say that was the most powerful intimidation I ever experienced. He knew he was a fucking lion!

That is the power, through this process, I am slowly gaining. Knowing unapologetically who the fuck I am. Not laced with insecurity and ego, but a gentle yet powerful love for myself, my life, and my God-given abilities.

My story, although dark and grim at times, was written mostly by my doing. If I were to place blame and culpability on others, I would continue to be powerless and another victim. I would remain immobile, malnourished, and ignored like the very baby I was born to in this world. My burdens and pains had become too much for me. I wanted them gone before it forced me to the worst alternative.

So I had to set my intention. What was it that I truly wanted to accomplish? Well, I wanted my pain to be gone and rid myself of victimizing patterns that were hugely inhibiting my progress and growth in this world.

I then had to identify, research and discover. Remember? I had to find out exactly what were all those major traumatic events in my life that affected me and my inner child so deeply. I had to open doors to a pile of skeletons I didn't really ever want to visit again, even though I knew they were there.

I had to feel into the pain and the hurt to help me understand better other related pain that manifested throughout my life. I was then able to ask myself if I was addicted to that pain in one way or another. How difficult was it going to be to let go? Was I alone with this sort of pain, or are there others out there that carry this yoke as well? If so, would I allow myself to open up and hear their stories, and would I be courageous enough to share mine?

I could then look back and take responsibility for my errors, my faults, and my failures. Accountability is very empowering when your ego is no longer in the way. This isn't hollow self-blame, but a noble act of self-responsibility and knowledge of where you know you fucked up.

Finally, permission. You outrightly give yourself permission to heal and permission to move forward. This simple mantra will empower you to move from where you once thought you were immovable.

I GIVE MYSELF PERMISSION TO HEAL AND MOVE FORWARD.

You will give yourself allowance and space to grow spiritually, mentally, and emotionally by ways you once thought dormant or nonexistent.

No matter what has occurred in your life, you do have divine power within you to change and correct your path, but you must do the work! You must awaken the true Warrior within you! You can no longer be a victim and cast blame to feed your ego. Throw your ego aside. Step into the unknown of finding your true self once again. Change your perspective and change your mind.

There is not one right path or one set of tools to take upon this work. The techniques I used to work through my pain that worked for me might not be right for you. But the ability to be persistent and undaunted by life's setbacks will prove fruitful.

No longer numb yourself away from your true purpose with vices and harmful drugs. It is time to accept yourself as you are right here and now. And then begin the work to create what you only imagined you could be.

I implore you to take a step into the unknown. For the first time in your life, I ask that you lean in and learn to trust. Find the inherent trust you have deep within you, and you will find a profound knowledge of power and love you have never before experienced!

Do the work! And become the WARRIOR!

CLOSING REMARKS

I want all to know I shared these words and my story not at all to look like a martyr nor a victim but merely a broken man who found his inherent power through self-healing and continuous intention to get better through very arduous work and discipline.

This is simply the roadmap I had to uncover for myself. Please do not assume I am painless or without trauma, for that would be false. I am simply a man who knows my pain, knows my trauma, knows who I am, and most importantly, I know my power.

Before, I was powerless, hopeless, and a victim. I have now stepped into my power through this work, with the ability to recognize and see my triggers that make me spiral off my path, and I know how to redirect a negative trajectory.

I also know I am the villain in possibly more than one person's story. I have hurt, let down, and disappointed people before, just as we all have. I have made a conscious effort to make many of those wrongs right, and for the rest, the opportunity has yet to present itself.

Out of all the accomplishments I am most proud in my life and of all the greatest gifts I have received, self-healing is by far my number one greatest achievement—next to my daughter—because not one damn person did it for me. I did it! And I was blessed by so many angels sent to me in human form that helped me along the way.

APPRECIATION

In my endless search for belonging and a sense of purpose, although not acknowledged until later in my life, I am now able to marvel in an unaltered state of gratitude for what has transpired in my life. I was given to parents who loved me so deeply and treated me no differently than if I was their very own. And looking back, they probably spoiled me more than the rest of my siblings.

I lost my mother in March of 2017 to cancer. She was a woman who loved me exactly like I needed to be loved and never allowed me to feel unwanted. She would always remind me of when she adopted me, how hungry and sad I was, and she did everything to fatten me up and make me happy. She did just that. Her strength and toughness are and will forever be within me.

I'm grateful for a father who was my biggest fan. He never missed a practice or a game. He taught me the importance of always being there for family no matter what. To never be afraid of letting anyone know how much you love and care for them. He stood toe-to-toe with any bully whoever hurt me, including their parents. He is a true definition of justice. He will forever be my hero.

To each of my siblings, thank you for loving me and being there for me. Whether it was just a hot meal, or a shoulder to cry on, you are my heroes and lifeblood.

Although raised in a culture with little or no acceptance, I am grateful for my friends who were and have always been there for me, no matter the circumstances. I attribute my perseverance, love, and support to each of you! Thank you for seeing and accepting me.

To my Queen, who has ridden this wave of uncertainty and darkness, even when there was no light to be seen, you still never give up on me. You pushed me to be great and saw my higher self when I never knew it even existed. You are my grace and my Warrior. I will love you forever!

And lastly to my beautiful daughter. You are a young queen in the making. Your eyes light my soul, and your laugh brings me more joy than I have ever experienced. You have given me purpose and filled my heart with more love than I knew I was capable of having. Watching you grow is my life's honor.

REFERENCES

Child Trends. (2016, February 23). *Parental Depression: A Multigenerational Threat.* https://www.childtrends.org/blog/ parental-depression-a-multigenerationalthreat

Hendricksen, E. (2016, October 20). Self-Injury: 4 Reasons People Cut and What To Do. *Psychology Today.* https:// www.psychologytoday.com/ us/blog/emotional-freedom/ 201007/the-health-benefits-tears? Amp

Kellermann, N.P. (2013). Epigenetic transmission of Holocaust Trauma: Can nightmares be inherited? *The Israel journal of psychiatry and related sciences.* https:// www.semanticscholar.org/ paper/Epigenetic-transmissionof-Holocaust-trauma% 3A-can-be Kellermann/ 7e9c87ca5e4823ed600dac4c 8a3bcccd5de17ff2?p2df

Orloff, J. (2010, July 27). The Health Benefit of Tears. *Psychology Today.* https:// www.psychologytoday.com/ us/blog/emotional-freedom/ 201007/the-health-benefits-tears? Amp

Pierre, J. (2018, September 5). Why Has America Become So Divided? *Psychology Today.* https:// www.psychologytoday.com/ us/blog/psych-unseen/ 201809/why-has-america-becomeso-divided?amp

Seupel, C.W. (2015, March 25). Blocking the Paths to Suicide. *The New York Times.* https:// www.nytimes.com/ 2015/03/10/health/blocking-thepaths-to-suicide.html

Smith, K. (2018, November 18). Reactive Attachment Disorder: Causes, Symptoms and Treatment. *Psycom.* https://www.psycom.net/ reactive-attachment-disorder